D0667841

AFTER
THE STROKE

Golden Age Books
Perspective on Aging

Series Editor: Steven L. Mitchell

AFTER
THE STROKE

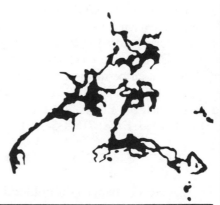

Coping with America's Third Leading Cause of Death

EVELYN SHIRK

PROMETHEUS BOOKS

Buffalo, New York

Published 1991 by Prometheus Books

95 94 93 92 91   5 4 3 2 1

Library of Congress Cataloging-in-Publication Data

Shirk, Evelyn Urban.
    After the stroke: coping with America's third leading cause of death.
        p.   cm.—(Golden age books)
    ISBN 0-87975-693-4 (cloth)—ISBN 0-87975-694-2 (pbk.)
    1. Cerebrovascular disease—Popular works. I. Title. II. Series.
RC388.5.S475   1991
616.8′1—dc20   91-3902
                                                                        CIP

Printed in the United States of America on acid-free paper.

"Nativity, once in the main of light,
Crawls to maturity, wherewith being crown'd
Crooked eclipses 'gainst his glory fight"

Shakespeare
from Sonnet XL

For Jay—and his fellow sufferers

"It's all I have to bring today
This and my heart beside . . .
This, and my heart, and all the fields,
And all the meadows wide"

Emily Dickinson*

---

*Introductory poem to Part Three, "Love," from *Poems of Emily Dickinson,* edited by Martha Dickinson Bianchi and Alfred Leate Hampton, New York: Little, Brown & Co., 1944

Foreword

Stephen Richmond, M.D.

Strokes can affect their victims in various ways. Some are relatively mild, leaving the individual with few, if any, lasting effects. Others, however, can be quite debilitating, rendering the person wholly or partially incapacitated.

The subject of this fascinating book was a leading scholar who succumbed to a tragic series of strokes, the cumulative effect of which left him physically handicapped and deprived of the ability to speak and write. Two essential tools of his personal and professional life were gone forever.

I met Jay and Evelyn after they had suffered through his first stroke and the ordeal of rehabilitation. The next few years were difficult for both of them. Jay was aware of many of the changes taking place within him, and he knew he was helpless to alter the course of events. I was inspired by the quiet dignity that fortified Jay year after year as he faced setbacks and struggled with disappointment.

Throughout my career, I have watched many patients confront the disabling aftermath of stroke. Medicine can often ease the physical discomfort associated with such conditions, but perhaps most painful of all is the mental anguish that stroke victims experience when faced with prolonged incapacity. It must have been incredibly frustrating for Jay, a man whose academic accomplishments were considerable, not only to lose his ability to communicate but to find himself unable to perform the most basic of tasks without assistance.

I marvel at Evelyn's strength as she took responsibility for Jay's care in their home. The many complications and obstacles she describes will give readers compelling, often poignant insight into the extraordinary effort required to care for a severely disabled individual. Her love and caring spirit fills each page as she chronicles their arduous seventeen-year journey punctuated by uncertainty, fear, and intense apprehension.

After Jay died, I learned that he was the author of two books I had studied during my freshman year of college. I remembered being impressed by these scholarly works. How ironic that years later I would be helping to care for this man. It was distressing to compare Jay the author with Jay the patient, but his efforts, and those of Evelyn, to retain personal dignity throughout their shared ordeal are inspiring.

Contents

1

The Starting Bell (1974)

The car slowed with the steepness of the hill that led to the little cottage by the lake. My husband, Jay, and I had opted to exchange the typically welcome income from summer teaching at the university for the experience of Vermont's luxuriant beauty. Its peaceful environment— enlivened by the sounds of insects, the lowing of cows, the arrogant "caw" of the crow and the hauntingly complicated song of the hermit thrush as it emerges from the depths of the forests at sunset—seemed to calm city-jangled nerves and to replenish vital energies. We invested the only money either of us had ever inherited in the little lakeside hideaway, to provide ourselves the recreation of swimming and boating. No sooner had we taken possession than it became ironically clear that our summers were too short to care for or enjoy the advantages of two homes. In both cases the houses and land required considerable attention and repair, and the new acquisition radically reduced our time for recreation at either site. We solved the problem by renting it out or loaning it to friends. We spent our summers at our old farm in the mountains of New England.

A colleague had given us, as a wedding present, a two weeks' stay at his antique farm in Vermont. We fell in love with the house and the state, spending our first two summers together searching for and finally finding our own mountain-top retreat. It was in such serious disrepair that it took a number of years to make it comfortably habitable. Our deepening relationship was cemented by doing most of the work ourselves, aided by the assorted jacks-of-all-trades which a Vermont village provides. Of course, none of this luxury would have been possible for two newly hired and impoverished young instructors had it not been for a continuous and very adequate stream of royalties from one of Jay's first and most successful books. In a playful mood, I covered the holes and falling plaster in Jay's study with a "wallpaper" of its galley proofs. These early years were exuberant, hardworking, and blissful. We spent our summer months every year in "The House that Royalties Rebuilt," punctuating our writing with home repair: the former activity seemed to season the latter with zest, and vice versa. We had made the right choice and we knew it.

Vermont was the place we longed for: to organize our thoughts, to contemplate their meanings, and to capture them in words. Somehow all that came effortlessly in such a tranquil setting. While we wrote in very different ways about very different topics and each spent much time in personal isolation, we shared the results of our efforts and joined in the common tasks of home-owning.

As the car rounded the top of the hill, the lake came unexpectedly into shimmering view. Who would have thought to find a lake nestled in a revine on top of a mountain? But Vermont was full of the unexpected. I was reassured. The little lake was still reliably there.

Expectation mounted as we drove a winding dirt road decorated by nature with colorful wild flowers and surrounded by untamed woods. The cottage soon came into view through a tangled wilderness of overgrown weeds and grass. I could feel Jay's anger surge as he surveyed the situation. I had not been married to him for over thirty years without knowing that he turned disappointment into fury toward whomever he believed to be the cause. The dock rested on the beach, the boats were upside down on the woodpile and chained to a tree, and the little garden looked forlorn from inattention. "Evelyn, I'll bet that the plumbing hasn't been reconnected!" Jay muttered angrily. His mood was not in harmony with mine, which was radiant with enthusiasm for the place. For me, these were disappointing facts but they would be remedied in due time. But Jay's expectations were frustrated and his annoyance mounted.

Upon returning to our farm, Jay unexpectedly asked, "Do you think I'm dragging my right leg? It doesn't feel right. It doesn't do what I want it to." He walked across the room so I could observe him: it was obvious that Jay *was* "dragging" his leg. His was a slurred walk, like slurred speech, in that it didn't come off with precision and there was some delay in his usual briskness. Perhaps he strained it going over the lake bank to the water. As if he had been reading my mind, Jay added, "And what's more, I can't say 'f.' " As he pronounced it I noticed that it didn't sound like his usual precise enunciation. It was as off-beat as a lisp.

The two symptoms joined in my understanding, and a feeling of dread came over me. The speech defect, minor as it was, brought back the memory of my mother, who crumpled to the floor in front of the refrigerator while she, my father, and I were enjoying a midnight snack. She had been stricken by something they called an "embolism" but eventually named a "stroke," about which I had some vague second-hand knowledge but had never before observed.

Disbelief, fear, and a need to repudiate the evidence Jay was presenting began to overtake me. Something was threatening Jay's BRAIN, and he was a man for whom inquiry and reasoning were not only his life's work but his deepest loves. I rushed to call our local doctor, who was reassuringly calm.

"I think he's had a 'transient ischemic attack,' " the term for a tiny, temporary stroke—a sort of sampler.

I latched onto the word "transient" and felt better. "Could it happen again? Does one attack predict another?" I asked.

The doctor likened the attack to being hit by a bolt of lightning, with the chances of recurrence being remote. But from the way he put it, I wasn't reassured.

"Come in tomorrow before you leave for the city," he said.

Jay's symptoms caused panic to hit, but I didn't show it. As I reflect on it, I can see certain advantages to having my expression of feelings tightly reined. For one thing, whatever fears there may be are more relieved by silence than by hollering, crying, and verbal outbursts. My own silence causes me to concentrate on whatever action seems necessary, and the action itself tends to syphon off anxiety, using its force for action. Second, my personal control often tends to reduce fear and tension in others by turning their attention away from their own hurt and toward the help that is being given.

However, there is an unfortunate flip side of this coin, namely, the two types of responses that emotional restraint elicits from on-lookers: some see me as "callous" and incapable of feeling, while sympathetic friends consider me "strong," "brave," and "able." Neither group fully understands the emotional dynamism involved.

The next morning the doctor recommended that Jay have a complete physical examination by specialists. Then he added, "Why not let your wife drive the long trip?" as a sort of suggestive prescription.

I gathered that another attack wasn't entirely out of the question. Besides, I knew not only that this unexpected physical event was different from any Jay had had before but that it was infinitely more ominous. Whether this was a "minor" or a "major" stroke, such as my mother's, didn't really matter. (It had caught her in the middle of a sentence and decreed that she would never speak again.)

During the tension-filled trip of seven hours, I contemplated what I should do if Jay were to have another attack while at the wheel. (He obviously did not choose to take the doctor's advice and allow me to drive.) I sat crosslegged in such a manner that my right foot could make contact with the brake in the event he unexpectedly slumped over.

All along I had remained "poker-faced," quiet, and motionless. My early childhood was responsible for this flat outward response to emotion, regardless of what might be going on inside me. "Make no noise" was the daily command from our overworked housekeeper. My mother, always in frail health because of heart problems stemming from a childhood bout with rheumatic fever, was typically ill and had taken to her bed. I was an only child until after my ninth birthday and there were no children on the block to play with; but even if there had been, there were no adults with time enough to watch over our play. Before starting school I was more or less confined to my room to amuse myself with toys and my beloved little victrola, which was always in use and always set on low volume. Early on, music seemed to possess me entirely and put me in an emotional world apart. Like most children, before I was able to read and write I responded well to music. I seemed already to know that music delivered intense feeling directly to the heart and the body, unadulterated by either thought or visual images. Jay and I shared this experience. Wherever we went, we made sure that the means to enjoy music were available, yet, ironically, neither of us played an instrument.

Being alone in my childhood, my imagination apparently burgeoned. According to my father, since I had no playmates, I invented them. I would warn him not to sit in a certain chair because "folks" were occupying it.

Like Alzheimer's disease, stroke affects the brain, though they are quite different ailments. Alzheimer's, for reasons not yet clear, distorts and disfigures brain cells, while stroke kills healthy cells by either drowning them in blood or starving them by cutting off the blood supply. Stroke occurs in a moment, whereas the symptoms of Alzheimer's accumulate so imperceptibly that neither the victim nor the family or companions recognize it for a long time. The effects of stroke are more or less reversible, but require considerable effort, courage, and patience, while those of Alzheimer's are not—at least not yet. Since the workings of the brain are inaccessible to ordinary perception (although the CAT scan, short for computerized axial topography,* can provide an image of some of them), the observer has some difficulty seeing and feeling the relation of cause to effect. In this sense, brain disorders are not comprehended in the way we come to understand a broken leg, a stomach ulcer, or a cancerous organ. While it is certainly true that the majority of us are medical laypersons who cannot be completely clear about the finer details of such ailments, nevertheless, we can in our own way— visually and viscerally—see, infer, and feel their effects as a loved one experiences them. We can co-feel where a stricken friend hurts: we can empathize with the person's fears and, with a bit of imagination, we can come to appreciate the possible progression of his or her ailment. But diseases of the brain baffle us, and they have throughout history. If we didn't already know that strokes are caused by internal brain damage, we would be hard pressed to connect the inability to move what appears to be an undamaged leg with some unseen malfunction taking place within the confines of the heavy bone structure of the skull. It isn't hard to sympathize with the medieval view that what we now know as brain ailments resulted from having become possessed by devils.

When I wasn't watching Jay's every move at the wheel, the same basic question kept creeping into my mind: "What *is* a stroke?" The answer can be found by taking a "look" at that part of the brain where the damage occurs. A few recollections from my biology classes reminded me that the brain is composed of two distinct sides or "hemispheres"— one on the right side of the head, the other on the left. Each hemisphere is said to govern one side of the physical actions of the body in addition

---

*The machine used for a CAT scan looks like a tunnel through which the patient is very slowly moved via a litter on a track. It takes many pictures of the brain from different levels, thus producing three-dimensional views. These permit doctors to identify both the location and the extent of the damage to the brain and to know the type and seriousness of the injury.

to governing very different functions of mind and thought. The surprising and perhaps unexpected fact is that the right side of the brain controls the *left* side of the body while the left side of the brain controls the *right* side of the body. It has always seemed to me that this remarkable cross-over, in some unclear way, assures the unification of the physical/ thinking organism into one interactive unit.

Jay was dragging his right foot, so the trouble—whatever it happened to be—was on the left side of his brain. This conclusion is further supported by the fact that the left side of the brain not only controls the right side of the body but also speech, logical reasoning, and mathematical ability—and Jay was unable to say "f." The right side of the brain is said to be responsible for another variety of reasoning, namely, that of imagination, artistic creation, fantasy, invention, and feeling.

These days it is fashionable to separate the imaginative hemisphere of the brain from its scientific, logical side. Yet it seems to me that these two types of thinking have some very intimate connections. Many scientific breakthroughs have been suggested by some highly poetic and imaginative thinking, or "thinking by analogy." We think by analogy when we view one thing as being "like" or suggestive of something else. Through recognizing common traits, we come to learn about one unknown thing by means of its likeness to something that we do know: for example, that electrons orbit around the nucleus of an atom like a "solar system" or that the willow tree "weeps" or that electricity "flows" like water. Logic and poetry are different types, different ways of thinking emerging from different brain locations, but I suspect that they often interrelate and spur each other on.

Looked at more closely, the two brain hemispheres consist of millions of cells arranged into groups, each of which controls specific tasks, such as speech, physical movement, organ functions, etc. The entire brain is nourished by a supply of blood that runs through small arteries, veins, vessels, and capillaries. Much of this blood comes to the brain through the large carotid arteries, which extend up either side of the neck in front of the ears.

Of the two kinds of strokes, the most typical is caused by a blood clot running loose in the victim's arteries or veins: it finds its way into a brain capillary, stops the flow of blood to that portion of the brain, and in so doing produces a stroke. Brain cells depending on that capillary for nutrition now have no food supply. As a result the cells "starve" and are no longer able to control the brain functions they once governed.

The second kind of stroke is caused either by a break or rupture in weakened capillary walls as they try to accommodate a slightly larger volume of blood or by a substantially larger blood flow exerting far too much pressure on relatively normal capillary walls. The result in either case is a breaking of the capillary wall with blood spilling over onto the surrounding brain cells. This, in turn, causes the cells to die.

Both kinds of strokes incapacitate brain cells, whose functions are thus interrupted. What we *see* with our eyes is that a leg can't work properly, but what caused this difficulty has happened in the brain. Today the CAT scan, used to analyze the brain, can provide doctors with an image of the exact location and extent of the brain damage— a tremendous asset for diagnosis, treatment, and prognosis.

The reason that the answer to the question "What happens in a stroke?" sometimes seems complicated is that "the" answer to this question turns out to be a series of answers to very different kinds of questions, each of which is equally important in understanding what has happened. Perhaps the first and more easily comprehended type of answer is the "physical" one. Considering the clot-type of stroke, it might be asked why there is fat residue in a person's blood in the first place. This, of course, brings us to the stomach and the gustatory time bomb it can hatch.

As we all know, Americans love their "juicy" fast food hamburgers, which are said to contain as much as one-third of their weight in fats. Then there are the "fries" soaked in fat. This is typically accompanied by a fat-laden milk shake or polished off by ice cream topped with chocolate, nuts, and whipped cream! Between meals there are, of course, potato chips, peanuts, and snacks of many sorts, all of which add not only more fat but provide substantial amounts of salt as their contribution to the impending trouble. Salt holds water in the blood thereby increasing its volume, causing it to struggle through pipes narrowed further by fat accumulations.

With stomachs filled with fat, the blood very shortly gives evidence of this fact by means of blood testing for "cholesterol." Cholesterol is nothing but a residue of fat in the blood. I shuttered as I recalled pictures of the arteries and veins of those who hadn't watched their diet. The layer of cholesterol reminded me of a cooked roast in a pan with the fat tending to rise to the top. As the pan juices are stirred, the fat clusters around the sides of the pan, making a sort of crust. This is precisely what happens in the arteries and veins. The fat globules begin to cluster along the sides of these vital tubes.

Meantime, the heart is pumping blood throughout the body. The fatter the body, the more flesh the heart has to service and hence the harder it has to pump. Furthermore, the more cholesterol that lines the arteries, the narrower the passageways become and the more force that must be exerted by the heart to pump the blood through this expanding network. The whole picture is rather like what happens as water courses through a garden hose. A large amount of water enters the hose from the spigot. If the nozzle is opened fully, the water runs through the hose easily and freely; but if the nozzle is narrowed, the velocity of the water increases to such an extent that we could water a lawn from twenty feet away. In much the same way, our blood is pushed through our arteries by the heart. As these arteries narrow with accumulated cholesterol, pressure begins to build up against the arterial walls. "High blood pressure" is a sign that the heart is not only working harder but that pressure against arterial walls is increasing thereby enhancing the chances that some fat will break off from an artery wall and enter the bloodstream. Many times these clumps are small enough to end up in a leg vein, where they are less destructive than when they end up in brain capillaries. At other times they are big enough to interfere with heart function (producing an "infarction") and cause death by "heart attack." The arteries, which supply the heart with oxygen-rich blood, could no longer deliver the supply that the heart needs to circulate throughout the body.

When such accumulations of fat build up in the carotid arteries, which serve the blood-supply needs of the brain, they are most likely (but not always) the cause of stroke. It takes but a small clot to damage the very tiny and sensitive brain cells that are connected to so many centers of action. Eleven years ago when Jay experienced his ischemic attack, the operation to "clean out" or remove the fat from the carotid arteries was considered a very risky operation. Patients too often died of clots that occurred as a result of the surgical procedure. No doctor mentioned this operation to me as a possible solution to Jay's problem or we might have considered it. On the other hand, knowing that the operation was especially risky, I am not at all sure that I would have favored it.

Furthermore, at the time, I had no idea that one stroke didn't finish the matter once and for all. A stroke had often been likened to being hit by lightning, which proverbially never strikes twice in the same place. Only in the light of a subsequent overview of the events of the years to follow would have permitted a rational judgment regarding the carotid artery operation. Hindsight is a wonderful deceiver. It distorts our sense of time, leading us to forget that the past was not and could not be identical to the present. We weren't in a position *then* to know what we know *now*.

At sixty-one and fifty-six respectively, Jay and I were no strangers to yearly check-ups. While I enjoyed good health, Jay's had always been more precarious. Back in the city, Jay's doctors began a complete reevaluation and found the usual culprits where both stroke and heart attack are concerned: namely, high blood pressure, a high cholesterol level, and a weight problem. Afterward we set about the required repair. Jay was given a diuretic to drain off the excessive liquid in his blood, thus reducing its volume. In the case of Jay's network of garden hose (arteries), the drug did much to turn down the volume of water pulsing through it. He was provided with a "heart medicine" to tone down his heartbeat, while a low-salt, low-fat diet was prescribed to reduce the amount of fat in his blood, a matter most Americans are far more aware of these days.

Necessity required that I learn how to cook for Jay's health without losing the attractive appearance and good taste of food. This was a crucial part of my caregiving role, especially since his enjoyment of food was always be one of Jay's most important sources of a sense of well-being and hope. To concentrate on "being on a diet," to be faced with unfamiliar food, or to find the dish unappetizing or taste-less can put a pall over what should be a "festive board." The job is not to simulate hospital food but to serve familiar and loved dishes —only this time with substitutes for forbidden ingredients. There are substitutes for eggs, cream, butter, and salt on the market these days and they are virtually undetectable. At least I have never had a dinner guest who caught on that he or she was eating an anti-stroke diet. I am not even sure that Jay knew much about these culinary maneuvers since we didn't discuss it. The less said about being deprived by a "diet," the better.

In the late seventies little or no emphasis was placed on developing exercise patterns, so no such program was suggested as an addition to Jay's daily routine. There is little doubt that with the addition of this type of regime, Jay might have improved even more, although once we Americans make a fad of something, we tend quickly to overdo it.

In the course of a year, Jay had lost almost forty pounds, his blood pressure had lowered to an acceptable level, and the amount of cholesterol in his blood dropped to a high normal. I was sure that the whole frightening episode was over and finished. Jay was pronounced in excellent health and medication was discontinued. We had won! We continued our dietary ways and I never stopped playing my game of devising satisfying and good-tasting food that held a special secret. I suppose I had just become accustomed to cooking that way. Life had returned to normal and the episode was more or less forgotten because the strange and short-lived disability seemed no longer threatening.

Yet I, for one, couldn't entirely dismiss the matter from my mind. My mother's lifelong crippling stroke formed a backdrop for my memories of Jay's attack. Questions about stroke continued to plague me. Perhaps this was because I didn't think to ask them at the time of my mother's terrifying seizure. I simply took for granted that she had an "embolism," whatever that was. Strange isn't it—if we can just give something a name, it settles our doubts, even if we haven't the foggiest notion about what the name means. At least it satisfies our urge to label things.

Furthermore, strange as it may seem, the questioner very often can't even put his or her question into words. While I had disturbing doubts about a lot of disconnected ideas, it was often difficult to find a group of words that would gather up all these loose ends and put them into a coherent question, the answer to which would put it all together for me.

Those to whom we look when answers are expected (e.g., doctors or teachers) have problems, too. After having taught for a number of years, I believe I have finally gained insight into the difficulties of answering questions in a way that would put an end to the puzzlement in a student's mind. The simpler and more direct the student's question, the more difficult it is to answer, simply because the "authority" possesses such a wealth of interconnected knowledge and insight that clear, easily contructed answers are difficult to assemble. Such questions as "What is Fascism?" or "Why does music 'send' us?" or "How do we really know that something is true?" or "What really happens in a stroke?" are enough to drive the would-be respondent to despair. Responses to questions like these are intricate patterns of distinct *types* of answers each of which is part of a larger whole.

I was sufficiently aware of this problem to be reticent about asking a physician such questions. I knew that the request for more information was an imposition on a doctor's time and patience, and often it put quite a tax on whatever skills he had in selecting the most useful ideas from his memory and putting them into words that a layperson, like me, would understand without the need for further elaboration. But now that Jay had been threatened by this mysterious illness and I was already older and more brash, I began to use my personal medical visits ever so subtlely to interrogate my doctor(s) regarding stroke. It helped. And I was also lucky enough to have another source of information: one of my good friends and colleagues at the University was its leading senior physiologist. For years we had many good conversations regarding a variety of medical topics, and my questions here were no exception. Always the teacher, he enjoyed answering my inept questions, while I was grateful for someone who was open to my many expressions of utter ignorance.

As I expected, the question "What causes stroke?" is indeed many-sided. Of course, there was the physical-mechanical side of it: the high blood pressure, the weight problems, and the presence of excess fat in the blood. But this account does not answer how brain damage can not only incapacitate its own thinking but can also immobilize remote parts of the body. To understand this aspect of stroke involves picturing the brain as a massive switchboard that sends messages throughout the body and receives messages from countless sources.

All of our senses send messages to the brain with regard to what is happening both in the world "inside" and the world "outside." The body tells the brain, "I am hungry," "I am sleepy," or "I am in pain," etc.; the brain receives these messages and responds with appropriate biological reactions. Or the brain will receive a message from the olfactory sense that something is burning in the kitchen and, in response, come up with the command, "Go find the source of the smoke and put it out." The command simultaneously sends a message to the muscles of the legs, back, and abdomen to accomplish the task of getting up and walking. Of course, the habits gained by muscles in continuing to get up and walk helps to accelerate the activity and make the action more accurate. The toddler trying to walk has not yet gained the habitual nerve paths that will later permit him to do such things with ease and without thinking. But for both toddler and adult, the brain transmits its command to the muscles. Needless to say, if the brain cells controling the muscles are damaged, the brain cannot transmit the message. Without receiving a message, the legs, back, and abdomen remain inert.

The great scientific discoveries since the eighteenth century regarding electricity and electromagnetism—what it is and how it can be generated, used, transmitted, and stored—have done much to further our understanding of the brain as a center of electrical impulses or "brain waves," which can be analyzed and measured and in terms of which, these days, we determine whether a person is "dead."

Our understanding of electricity has also brought about a number of technological benefits: from the telephone to facsimile machines, from incandescent lighting to the transistor. It has helped provide an abundant supply of household appliances that can accomplish almost all of our household tasks. And it also helped make possible office equipment and the computer. It is the computer which, far and away, reminds us of, and teaches us about, the way that the human brain operates. The brain has been imaged as a computer, masterminding not only our physical life but our intellectual one as well. The basic logic underlying a computer's ability to "reason" bears a striking resemblance to the way in which we do a variety of reasoning tasks and the way in which we store and recall data from our "memory banks." The computer "thinks" logically in the sense that it can "recognize" messages and can, by using its stored data, "respond" to certain questions posed to it by using that data. The human brain does precisely this.

Perhaps the greatest advantage of the computer over the human brain is the incredible speed with which it can sort through data to find the needed facts and the incredible range and speed of its ability to perform various mathematical and logical operations with those facts. Consider the bank of computers in NASA's "Mission Control" room: it "reports" on every programmed facet in the infinitely complex network of actions and reactions going on within and around the spacecraft. All mechanical events are electronically transmitted to the master computers, which then report "go ahead" or "danger." If "danger," human brains interact with the computer "brains" to concoct a "menu" of possible moves to be made in order to rectify the reported difficulties. NASA's computers are programmed to send correcting messages to the machinery, after which both astronauts and computers report back regarding whether the remedy was successful. This is suggestive of the way doctors and patients interact to produce a diagnosis and a plan of action for a remedy.

Along these same lines, when we are swimming and notice a sting ray nearby, the brain instantly calls for adrenalin to be sent to the muscles to enable a speedy getaway. If we are lost in a forest, the brain marshals data from our "memory banks" to suggest possible solutions to the problem of how to find recognizable ground. It is the computer brain that corrects our efforts to reach for and grasp a glass without spilling or dropping it. It is the computer brain that calculates and corrects for the pitcher's throw so that he can get the ball correctly over the plate at the proper speed. It is the computer brain that monitors our walking. And if we start to fall, it magnanimously works to prevent or ameliorate the accident.

In computerese, a stroke is a bug in the machine and a glitch in its performance—a malfunction in its mechanical guts. A stroke interferes with message exchange between the brain center's command-control and muscular obedience. A stroke can also disrupt and even black out parts of the brain's memory bank, which results in our inability to do mathematical operations should it hit those sectors in the brain, or it can cause loss of the ability to recall familiar words as well as the ability to enunciate word sounds.

One question that intrigued me is just how these messages between brain and body are conveyed: What serves as the "wires"? This network is more difficult to develop an image of because we are not dealing solely with things extended in space or "body." Efforts to create a purely physical image of these message relays results in inaccuracies not unlike the belief that electricity is some liquid or "juice" that "flows through" wires. It's probably more accurate to say that electrical impulses coming from the brain often use a signal system of chemical languages to activate various muscles, glands, nerves, and organs to carry out its commands. The chemical languages or signals are rather like the special languages with which we program the computer. Suffice it to say that if the sending mechanisms of the brain are damaged, the messages necessary to control physical functions cannot be sent and the body remains inert.

The similarity of the human brain to a computer need not be mind-boggling. Just remember that we humans program computers with the laws and traits of our own logic. We make the computer in our own image and program it to answer the questions we want it to answer. It is not as if the computer arises out of nowhere and, lo and behold, it is like our own brain. Rather, since we humans made the computer, we constructed it in such a way that we can interact with it and become its "companion." The "miracle" is not that the computer is so much like the human brain but that it can perform human brain functions with infinitely greater speed and accuracy. Using the capabilities of electricity, our society has made a machine that extends our own abilities, thus giving us powers of control over our world that we never had before.

A computer, however, is not a brain. A brain is capable of certain functions and capabilities that a computer cannot manage. For example, a brain can think "analogically," that is, it can "see" and "feel" similarities between two things. In so doing, it can understand one thing by means of its knowledge of another. "Analogical" thinking is not "illogical" or nonsensical but a different kind of thinking. It does not violate science and logic but simply operates using another kind of logic, which comes from the senses and feelings rather than from rules of inference. When the poetess proclaims her "lifetime folding up" or that she would "taste eternity" or was "stroking the melody" or could "hide in a flower" we take her to be suggestively arousing feelings and thoughts by showing us the familiar in a new and striking way. This is precisely what creative scientists do when they see a similarity between an atom of carbon and the "architecture" of the heavens, and when they conclude that the entire universe of matter, both small and large, is built on the same electromagnetic constellation plan.

A second sample of the differences between a human brain and a computer is that while the computer's reasoning can always be translated into words, the human brain can "reason" nonverbally, as does the composer when creating music and the painter when formulating a picture. Each reasons and makes selections that go into the work of art in terms of imagined sound, tone, beat and color, design, balance, and arrangement. These are selected on the basis of their accompaniment of feeling and emotion. The computer does not have hopes, longings, elations, or sorrows, hence it can never duplicate the human brain's expression of such things. While computer-generated poetry, painting, and music can interest and amuse, it hardly touches the wellspring of human feeling.

A third sample of the functions that only the human brain can perform are those we call "empathizing" or "co-feeling" with others. It is this very ability that permits us to "appreciate" and "enjoy" the thing called "art" in the first place. The computer can hardly "sympathize" with our anger and anguish when it is "down" and we are frustrated. Nor can it duplicate our joy when it predicts large business profits.

A fourth sample brings us to perhaps the most important difference of all, namely, that the human brain can evaluate the ethical worth (or lack of it) of our actions. While, like the brain, it can determine which answers are financially sound and cost-effective, it cannot add the further dimenson of whether those answers are "fair," "kind," and "humanly decent." It is this type of thinking that makes us responsive to the claims and needs of others and enables us to move to alleviate the plight of the sick, the old, the endangered, and the economically enslaved. It is this kind of thinking that makes us "caregivers." And it is this kind of thinking that determines what victims do with their plight when they evaluate it. They can conclude that their illness robs their life of all value and hence give up and succumb to it, or they can valiantly fight their infirmities in order to either overcome them or make ingenious adaptations. It is because of this value dimension pervading human thinking that the job of the caregiver is to pay special attention to the victim's level of optimism, sense of well-being, and will to live. It is not enough to feed, wash, change bandages, etc. At the heart of the enterprise is being especially aware of the person's images, fantasies, feelings, and evaluations—none of which the computer brain can handle.

2

The First Knock-Down Blow (1979)

The department meeting had gone well: I was satisfied that we had made some progress with curricular development. Suddenly the secretary interrupted. There was a call for me from State University. Did I know where the Professor was? He had not met his classes that day, nor had he called!

I stood speechless. Thoughts tumbled over questions in such a massive pile-up that I found a quick response impossible. A feeling of dread and foreboding was creeping over me. What had happened? I couldn't remember when Jay had last missed a day of classes. No ordinary illness or mishap would have prevented him from notifying his students in order to spare them inconvenience. It simply was not in Jay's nature to renege on his obligations. Had he become ill at home or had he had an accident on the road? I would only know which was the correct scenario if could just locate his station wagon. If it was parked in the driveway, he was still at home; but if it wasn't there then whatever happened occurred on the road. I grabbed my coat. I had to find out which it was, and fast! Our department secretary, who unpretentiously called herself "M. F.," put on her coat. "I am going with you," she said. Her decisiveness conjured up foreboding.

Never was the trip home longer. Anxiety was eating away at me. As I rounded the final corner, our driveway came into view. And there stood the wagon, mutely but eloquently delivering its silent message.

M. F. was beside me at the door as I fumbled and then dropped the house keys. "I can't put it in the lock," I said. She replied imperiously, "Put the key in the lock and turn it!" As I entered, I caught a glimpse of our dog, Flecky, streaking up and down the stairs in apparent frenzy but I didn't hear her message. A quick circle around the first floor revealed nothing. We raced up the stairs with the frantic dog under foot. There, on the floor in his library, beside his reading chair, was Jay, lying on his right side with his right arm under him. Since he was not yet dressed for work in his usual immaculate fashion and since I knew that he typically left at eleven A.M., he must have been stricken between ten and eleven. He had been on the floor in this position, unable to move, for nearly seven hours. I gathered, and he later affirmed, that the dog never left his side but lay beside him, ears cocked, muzzle on Jay's outstretched hand, awaiting my return. She "knew" that he was in trouble.

I rushed to Jay's side. His eyes were open and he was apparently conscious, but he didn't seem to be able to speak: he didn't utter a sound, although he seemed to know me. Panic hit. I propped him up and cradled him in my arms while M. F. rushed to call the police. It wasn't long before he was strapped to a chair, carried downstairs and bundled onto a stretcher. For the first time—but by no means the last—I followed an ambulance.

It was a long night of paper signing and apprehension and I didn't seem to be able to do anything effectively, I didn't know what to do or how to do it. Whatever "stunned" means, I think I was.

"It's a stroke, on the right side," they announced. Jay lay in the Emergency Room, his eyes closed and his forehead beaded with sweat. No, they couldn't tell me how serious it was or whether he would ever speak again. That could only be determined by a CAT scan and, later on, by a long and arduous process of testing his various capacities in order to identify the effected areas.

A stroke on the right side. It figured. He was lying on his right side. He must have gotten up from his chair when the clot hit him, at which point his right leg must have collapsed under him and he went crashing to the floor. The right foot was the one he had dragged five years previously at the lake! I wondered whether his right arm had been hurt since he had been lying on it for so many hours; the circulation in that arm must have been severely constricted. My fears were later borne out.

It was one A.M. when M. F. and I returned to the house and

sat quietly in the kitchen. I served her the dinner I had prepared for Jay. I was beyond hunger.

When I arrived for my early class, not too many hours later, M. F. was already at work. We just looked at one another in silence. She had put her hand over mine as I leaned on her desk. My gratitude for all her help that night was not expressible in ordinary words, although poetry or music might have been able to suggest my feeling.

It wasn't long before colleagues and close friends called and came to bring comfort, compassion, and the warmth of solicitude. An academic community is really a small town with many close-knit human connections, across many intellectual disciplines. So satisfying are some of these relationships that there seems to be little need and, ruefully, less time, for many "outside" connections.

Two months of hospital regime followed. It had indeed been a major stroke involving Jay's speech center, his right arm, and his right leg. We didn't yet know that his mathematical brain had also been severely damaged, but in due time every one of his capacities was tested— arms, legs, hearing, seeing, speaking—and his ability to read and write came under arduous scrutiny.

Within several weeks, Jay began to speak again, but it came with difficulty. His speech was hesistant and he seemed to struggle to find words. I began to notice that something remarkable was happening. He was not speaking in his usual fashion and didn't sound like himself. He seemed to be using substitute words—odd phrases and synonyms— for what he wanted to say. Then it dawned on me: Jay was speaking poetry! Poetry is, after all, a startling and unique way of expressing thoughts and feelings which nonpoets put into flat prose. The layers of meaning to be found in poetry cannot be expressed in prose, which aims at expressing its content unambiguously and single-mindedly, and avoiding words and phrases that would open the door to many individual, feeling-clad meanings. Prose constricts, in order to achieve accuracy of interpretation, while poetry freely opens doors in order to invite layers of personal meaning to be encountered.

Jay had always loved words and enjoyed playing with them. But he exalted in poetic expression. His speech was now a beautiful and haunting kind of communication by poetic analogy. So often in the past, his account of an event would be punctuated by remembered lines from Dunne, Blake, Wordsworth, Coleridge, or the Bible. He had written a book on poetry several years previously and now his illness seemed to have made him a poet by necessity!

On the other hand, something seemed to have happened to his understanding of events and their implications. One day I found him in a lounge where he had been put to watch television. I joined him to watch and keep track of the Three-Mile Island impending nuclear disaster. Much to my astonishment he didn't seem to understand what was happening or the danger it posed to people and to the fertile Pennsylvania countryside. Even my concern for our daughter, who was living some fifty miles from the scene, brought no response. He commented, "Daisies in the field but the big cylinders rule over them." Apparently he was unable to comprehend the meaning and the dangers inherent in a meltdown but could only see the contrast between the beauty of the land and the ugliness of the reactors. (I had, by this time, become able to decipher his extemporaneous poetry.)

Yet Jay could read. Among the tests to determine which capacities were lost was a presentation of the daily newspaper and a command to read the headlines. Whether he understood what he read was more difficult to discern. I rather think now that his ineptitude with current events was because he had already been out of the world for almost two months. That seemed to be borne out by the fact that he clearly understood the implications of close, homey things.

I was beginning to realize that I was both lonely for Jay's companionship and afraid of being in the house alone. I had been interlaced with a family since I was born and had moved easily from that to marriage. It was an unexpected and intimidating shock to confront our home's dark facade at night. Even the dog's enthusiastic greeting failed to dispel my sense of physical isolation and psychic abandonment. One night, listening to radio news, I learned that a couple we had known for years had been murdered in their beds. I ordered a lighted dial phone for my bedroom so that I could call the police from under the covers! Nor could I persuade the habit-bound dog to substitute my bedroom for her accustomed bed in the basement. Jay understood my fears. "You must keep an open house," he said, "and generously scatter brightness around." (Translation: "Keep all of the inside doors open and turn on the lights here and there.")

Apparently I had become dependent on Jay's presence in ways I had not known. Despite the fact that we typically worked in our separate studies, two floors apart, he had nonetheless provided a "thereness," an assuring presence, always available, to be counted on. I was to discover my own loss of "wholeness" without him. As Plato's myth has it, I was longing for the "other half" to make me whole.

Furthermore, like so many other "independent" women, I discovered not only my previously hidden dependency but also my utter lack of "know-how" in dealing with the house's occasional illnesses and obstreperousness. I surely had never before encountered its bills and financial dealings, which Jay's absence now demanded of me. Mortgage payments and utility bills were a mystery. Jay had always managed these things, but now I was obliged to confront my abject ignorance and ineptitude. Jay's comment on my woes with the bills was, "Time will wait; you will slowly drift into satisfaction." (Translation: "Slow up! No hurry! You will learn to do these things in good time.") But I didn't "drift" so easily or so soon. Rudderless, I made my way through the maze of financial detail that he had managed for so long. In short, I felt a kind of insufficiency, which I am sure that not only women feel but men as well when illness, death, and even divorce separates them from a spouse. The marriage vow proclaims, "And the two shall become as one," thus predicting a kind of merging of personal boundaries, which makes even temporary separation uncomfortable.

Meanwhile, the hospital had determined which muscles and capacities the stroke had damaged, and set up both speech and physical therapies to help Jay recover some of his losses. In the meantime, I went to the many question-answering sessions, briefings, and exchanges of caregiving problems, which our county had provided for the husbands and wives of stroke patients. I read the pamphlets they handed out.

After two months in the hospital, the doctors felt that they had done as much as they could for Jay. They recommended that we apply to the Rusk Institute of Rehabilitation, about which I knew absolutely nothing. Jay's doctors applied to Rusk on his behalf but were not optimistic about immediate acceptance since Rusk's reputation was world-wide and the waiting list was long. But Jay's professional reputation and personal accomplishments must have aroused their interest. Apparently the Institute was curious how a stroke would affect a philosophy professor.

The doctor assigned to Jay's case at the Institute wanted to see his books and seemed especially interested in his language and modes of expression. I think that my comment that he now spoke only poetry had a special meaning for them. It did for me, too, as I refined my view that when his logical side could not comply in his search for words, Jay's brain transferred his request to its other side, the analogical side, and it was from there that he got the unusual poetic way of expressing himself.

Jay was accepted into the Rusk Institute immediately. Celebration was in order for the hope we now felt. He was taken by ambulette* and put into a room with two young men, each suffering irreversible paralysis. The first had dived into an empty swimming pool and broken his neck. The second had fallen off of a moving train and broken his back. Since neither was over twenty-one and both were never expected to walk again, Rusk set about teaching them how to establish and maintain a successful wheelchair life.

I began to see that tragedy was not entirely reserved for older adults, but I had not yet seen the children. On one occasion, an elevator door opened and I was confronted with ten or twelve miniature wheelchairs holding youngsters so distorted, disfigured, and disabled, without hands and some without legs or feet. Many had disfigured faces and some had their heads lolling on their shoulders because they could not hold them up. It was shattering and absolutely God-defying. I shall never forget that sight, because it put my own complaints regarding Jay's illness into sharp perspective.

The Rusk Institute is a large, bustling, many-storied establishment nestled by the East River in central Manhattan. It was apparently the first facility of its kind anywhere in the world. Dr. Rusk, a physician for the battle-injured troops of World War I, had come to the conclusion that not only physical incapacity due to various kinds of damage to the body but also damage to the governing brain was theoretically reversible. The brain was, after all, capable of making and finding new paths, bypasses, and detours to inert muscles. Furthermore, the brain had a remarkable and unique capacity: healthy brain cells could and do take over the duties of damaged and dead cells, almost as if nature itself recognized the prime importance of the brain and gave it not only the skull for protection but also the special privilege of being able to reestablish its regal control over the body.

Doctors and researchers at the Institute put this knowledge to practical use and developed the first tentative programs in physical medicine designed to rehabilitate the stricken. So successful were Rusk's efforts that out of them grew a new branch of medicine, "Physical Medicine," which has since became a medical specialty for some two thousand practitioners in this country in the last ten to twenty years. The conviction of the doctor of physical medicine is that physical disabilities arising

---

*A conveyance for wheelchairs, complete with ramp and chains to anchor the chair while in transit.

from whatever cause—car accidents, sports accidents, cerebral accidents such as stroke, and even the ailments of overzealous aerobic dancers— had a better-than-fair chance of being lessened or eradicted altogether by its innovative programs. With the increasing infatuation of the American public with the idea that regular exercise of one kind or another could strengthen heart muscles and prolong life, along with the idea that there can never be too much of a good thing, physical medicine has grown apace both in knowledge and skill.

Accompanying this medical advance was the development of a series of therapeutic techniques and support devices designed to accomplish these results. This was followed by an army of "physical therapists" trained to carry out the orders of the physicians. These included exercises, baths, and massages, as well as manual and electronic techniques designed to stimulate and rehabilitate the damaged areas of the body. I became especially interested in physical therapy and its practitioners, having had some rewarding personal experience with it.

I suspect that in all of medicine, physical therapy requires the greatest patience, persistence, and forebearance on the part of both patient and therapist. It also requires a never-failing optimism regarding a successful outcome, which seems to be continuously repudiated by equally persistent incapacities. Patients must be willing to concentrate their efforts on trying to overcome their afflictions, with all their heart and will, despite recurrent failure. Recovery is so gradual as to be almost imperceptible. As it inches along, the therapist spurs the patient on with praise, even though only an eighth of an inch of new movement occurs after two or three weeks of painstaking work. No dramatic breakthroughs here; no sudden reversals or surprises. Yet in most cases, movement does gradually begin to return. Only after weeks and months can one realize that remarkable progress has been made in reversing a muscle's inertia.

The Rusk Institute is a well-developed sample of the many-sided efforts made to bring muscles and the brain together to work toward repairing the damage. Jay's regime began with the doctors identifying his areas of incapacity and evaluating the extent of the stroke. An individualized program of treatment was designed and later outlined to him. Jay's day was divided into sections, each of which was devoted to isolating some side of his incapacity and working on it.

Bent on utilizing not only muscles but all types of interests, needs, and conditions of life, the Institute presented a wide array of activities and facilities to encourage patients to be active. There were sessions on all sorts of arts and crafts to bring hand muscles into operation: paper cutouts, bead stringing, painting, drawing, piano playing, and typing, depending on each patient's inclination. It boasted a greenhouse where gardening enthusiasts could use their hands in potting and tending plants. There was a complete kitchen for teaching wheelchair patients how to handle their needs: preparing food, cooking, feeding themselves, and tending to kitchen chores. A larger-than-life automobile was on hand to train patients in entering and exiting cars, and there were sessions on learning to drive again. The Institute even provided the services needed to outfit a particular patient's car for special physical needs. The staff even arranged new driving tests for those with specially equipped cars. The Rusk Institute provided every incentive for patients to continue to hope and hence to try even harder to reach agreed-upon goals. Apparently most continued to try, since many succeeded.

Under the Rusk roof, Jay progressed nicely: learning how to walk and manage stairs again, at first with the aid of a therapist, then with a cane, and finally by using the bannister. He reestablished his ability to turn on the shower and wash and dress himself. In two months he was able to enter a car with minimal aid and be brought back home without a nurse. After almost half a year of this grueling ordeal, Jay wept with joy and disbelief as he again crossed the threshold of the home he loved. He had beaten back the devils of despair and helplessness and was ready to take up life again.

A financial note to this first serious encounter with stroke is in order because it will then be possible to make some contrasts with later developments. Jay's stroke occurred two weeks before his sixty-fifth birthday. Since Medicare starts on the first day of the month in which one turns sixty-five, he was already on Medicare when we found him motionless on his study floor. Medicare was his first provider—and provide it did. During almost six months of care, both the hospital and the Rusk Institute took care of *all* paperwork, and Medicare, plus Jay's private insurance from State University, paid in full for every facet of his care. We never received a single bill. In short, we went financially unscathed—so far.

3

Time Out (1980–1981)

If Jay had made rapid progress at the Rusk Institute, he doubled his speed upon returning home. Delighted at being freed from Rusk's demanding schedule, he seemed to enjoy everything, from being able to listen to his Baroque music to reading the morning newspaper and savoring home-cooked food. Hope and eagerness to get going again were written all over him. We were hardly home a week before he proposed making our annual summer visit to Vermont! He wanted to take up his life again at exactly where it had been forcibly interrupted.

I had certain reservations about a trip that was long enough to warrant an overnight stay. I had not been with Jay long enough to determine his abilities and his stamina and I didn't know how much I would be called upon to do. I did realize, however, that most of the little things he had formerly done, such as walking the dog and registering at the motel, would now be added to my list. Furthermore, the uneven Vermont terrain would be treacherous for unstable legs. If Jay wanted to walk alone in the woods, as he usually did, could he make it?

In addition to these concerns, Jay had latent agoraphobia, which had shown itself now and then throughout his life. It surfaced during some previously disturbing experiences on the New England Thruway, which, in Vermont, typically rides the mountain tops. I felt sure that he would ask me to take the old, lowland route, which was too narrow and winding for our oversized station wagon, besides which it would take us through so many small towns that we'd never make good time arriving at our destination. It would take several hours longer, and I wanted to shorten the trip as much as possible. I was plainly nervous about my cargo: a recovering invalid and an over-eager dog that knew, by the looks of the baggage, she was on her way to her favorite spot.

Of course, Jay wanted to go the lowland route, if for no other reason than that his recent disablement had dredged up his earlier anxieties. I braced for the trip by reminding myself that since he was now at home and was so intensely eager to do many things, I would, in good time, have many more problems of this nature to worry about.

With my own anxiety bubbling over at the edges, we set out. It was the first time that Jay had ever ridden with me at the wheel. On all of our trips together, either I was his passenger or I followed him in my car. Jay's uneasiness began to show: he winced every time I passed a car, claiming that I passed too closely. On the other hand, he was equally agitated when I returned to the right side of the road. He'd whimper "Oh! Oh!" and grab the dashboard. Again he claimed that I was too close to the edge of the road. Shortly I began to discern what the trouble was. Jay had never before, during our long marriage, sat in the front passenger seat! He had never before seen or felt what driving from that vantage point was like and it all seemed very dangerous to him! I resolved on the spot to make all our young married friends aware of just how imperative it is that they should share responsibilities for financial matters, driving with the other partner as a passenger, and tending to the kitchen and providing the food. Specialization may be a great thing but it loses much of its charm when someone in the partnership gets sick.

Not unlike many other travelers, we had to stop along the way so Jay could use a bathroom. For stroke victims such needs not only come suddenly but with special urgency. I spotted a tiny public library in a "town" that, at first glance, appeared to consist of the library and one lone all-purpose store. But the library came first. Jay walked unsteadily to its door only to emerge somewhat crestfallen not long thereafter, and with an expression of resignation. He had been denied the key! I was furious. My first impulse was to have it out with the person responsible for such an outrage. But this would have taken time, and Jay's needs came first. I drove the car across the empty street to the "grocery" store where I knew from experience that a lavatory would be typically found somewhere in the back of the store, surrounded by soap powders. All of a sudden I realized *why* Jay had been denied! What else could an uncertain gait and slurred speech mean to an unimaginative stranger than that either Jay was drunk or drugged? I simply had become so accustomed to Jay's incapacities that I really didn't "notice" them any more. I remembered meeting someone whose face had been almost blown totally away by an explosion. At first I was entirely shocked, horrified, and dismayed; I didn't want to look at him, so great was my revulsion. But after I came to know him well, I no longer "saw" his disfigurement. It wasn't a shocking surprise any more. I debated, but only for a moment, about revealing my conclusion to Jay. His self-esteem was in much too precarious a state for such a revelation.

This time I took over the reins. We entered the store together and I introduced both Jay and myself and explained both the stroke and the need. Never was anyone more obliging and solicitous than that shopkeeper. "OF COURSE!" he said, offering his help if necessary. Nothing beats knowledge of the facts, I thought to myself—realizing that at the same time I had decided NOT to share with Jay my knowledge of why his request had been previously denied.

This somewhat troubled and pathetic story brings to mind another obstacle in the path of those of us who care for a stroke victim. Rule 1, which caregivers are typically given, is the admonition not to do too much for the patient who is in the throes of learning how to do for himself. Rule 2, of course, is to unobtrusively help the victim when that becomes obviously necessary. Those who want to help are thereby left with the obligation to decide which situation they face and hence whether or not to act. Following rules brings on a decision-dilemma since rules are always applied to particular situations and to the particular individuals in them. I consoled myself with the conviction that, should I make an error, I won't be the only one who has. Nor will I be the only one to regret, in retrospect, whatever decision had been made.

The summer went better than expected. Jay read, listened to music, and enjoyed the scenery. I had put my foot down heavily on his desire to roam the woods alone, with the dog, or even with me. Vermont woods tend to be laden with booby traps even for those who are young and agile.

It was during our vacation in Vermont that I asked Jay a mathematical question pertaining to some financial data I was responsible for.

"Don't ask ME", he said, "I can't even add two and two." And then he added, "Even writing my own name is like moving the Aegean Stables; it takes me half an hour to accomplish it."

All at once I remembered what they had told me at Rusk, but I guess I hadn't really digested the information. Suddenly Jay's disabilities and their implications came down on me heavily . . . too heavily to believe his assertion. I thought he might be exaggerating or even joking. Then I remembered what his doctor at the Institute had told me: "How arresting it is that his philosophical brain has escaped destruction while his mathematical brain has not." I realized that whatever reservations I had regarding my own mathematical abilities, I had to face the fact that financial matters were destined to be my responsibility in the future whether I liked the role or not.

When we returned to the city, our lawyer suggested that Jay give me a durable and complete power of attorney over all of his affairs. Jay eagerly agreed. *Someone* must take the responsibility for financial matters and for signing papers. This unrestricted power of attorney has come in handy on many occasions since.

Jay began to plan for an "experimental" seminar for his graduate students to be held in our family room at home during the fall term of 1979. He wanted to try his hand at teaching again before he returned to the University for the spring semester. Twelve students arrived, and from the animated conversation (for three and four hours at a time) emerging from the basement, I gathered that Jay had not only regained his full powers of speech but also his intellectual acumen. In pleasure and gratitude for this welcome turn of events, I became an absentee hostess, preparing refrigerated refreshments for the group the night before.

"Happiness" for me is often manifested by a certain amount of teasing and humor. After one of these "Cellar Ceminars," the students congregated in the kitchen to share pleasantries with me and to express appreciation for the food. On one of these delightful occasions, a student cornered me and asked hesitantly, "What were those green specks in the tuna mousse?" I suspected what he was thinking, and I simply couldn't resist. I put on a straight face, looked him right in the eye, and I said, "mold"! He blanched and I repented. Laughingly, I explained that it was parsley from my herb garden at the side of the house. Always the teacher, I explained that parsley fresh from the garden tends to retain the vivid green of its chlorophyll. Now, belatedly, I wish I had been able to sit in on these joyful and reassuring sessions, but my own teaching obligations interfered.

It was with considerable enthusiasm that we set about planning Jay's return to the University in spring of 1980. A limousine service was to drive Jay the thirty-five miles to and from the campus; a local taxi was lined up to take him from one part of the sprawling institution to another; and he was to be housed overnight at the local inn, which also served excellent meals. This way he could leave home on Wednesday morning, teach a seminar and counsel his students, stay at the inn overnight, teach a second seminar the next day, and be driven home immediately thereafter. The schedule was relatively easy and Jay was able to handle it all, including the steep stairs at the old inn. Despite the elaborate arrangements, there were no slip-ups.

It occurred to me that, despite his long, tough illness, Jay had missed only five weeks of classes the previous spring, barely putting a dent in his previously untouched sick-leave allowance. And he had returned to fulltime teaching a short nine months after his stroke! Surely he had made a remarkable recovery!

During this happy time, many of Jay's friends (and mine) came to visit, among them his chess-playing buddies. Jay had typically been the champion during the pre-stroke sessions. So fond was he of the game that many of my gifts to him were unusual and beautiful sets of chessmen. At one point I gave him "Boris," a computerized game with the machine as his opponent. Boris had a lively sense of humor and would flash some very snide remarks on the screen if it "sensed" that a particular move was foolhardy. Jay could now play chess without having to wait for human visitors! But for some reason, Jay didn't ask for Boris. When his chess-playing friend (who was also a mathematician) arrived, I brought out the board. Jay lost the game; in fact, he lost all of them! I had totally forgotten about his damaged mathematical brain and its close connection with chess-playing. I should have remembered this, and for a while I felt very guilty. And then Jay said, "I don't think that I am able to play chess any more." He said it with such deep regret that I secretly and sorrowfully put all of the chess paraphernalia away, where it has remained ever since.

4

Sparring (1982–1986)

Jay taught for two and a half years after his stroke, until the beginning of the spring term, 1982. At the age of sixty-eight he decided to retire. Jay felt he was speaking too slowly and this hampered his ability to teach, though I had not noticed any evidence of this. Furthermore, he continued to experience the typical chronic exhaustion of which stroke victims so often complain. He was *tired.* His students protested; at last they could take adequate notes!

The first two years of Jay's retirement brought an army of visitors. Sitting regally in his motorized chair, Jay received student friends; previous student friends, now employed; former colleagues; and assorted well-wishers.

Almost daily I would return from the University to find that I was destined to have impromptu guests for dinner. While I enjoyed conviviality and was grateful that Jay so much enjoyed his guests, it surely taxed my ability to be a good hostess and provider. Such things have to be planned, and these were not. Besides, I was tired and frequently faced a very busy evening at work in my study. Very shortly I learned how a dinner planned for two could be instantly expanded into a meal for three to six by appropriate additions.

We had time for, and interest now in, returning to our previous habits of planned entertaining. We visited old friends and they visited us for good dinners at home, followed by an evening of pleasant conversation.

41

Visits from our relatives, however, were scarce since we only had four. Our daughter lived several hundred miles away and was working in the media, which typically pays little attention to holidays or other opportunities for time off. Jay's sister and her husband, and his niece, were not geographically "near" either. Even this frenetically busy couple tolerated an hour and a half trip through dense traffic to spend an evening or two with us during the year.

In that same summer Jay succumbed to his anxiety in the passenger seat and decided that he would not accompany me to Vermont. He had already turned his driver's license back to the state on the grounds that his stroke had made him unsure of his judgment of distance. The state responded with a "Certificate of Commendation" for his good sense. Disappointed, and even a bit frightened, I sorrowfully remembered our caravan-type trips with both cars. It went without saying that Jay would lead. For years we did this without ever losing one another, because Jay had a solution that was unfailingly effective. Should a car come between us, Jay would slow down dramatically. Immediately, the offending driver would pass Jay, and we would once again be "vehicularly reunited," as he put it.

I prepared for my trip alone. I was going not particularly for pleasure but because a house without inhabitants for many months has a tendency to develop some ailments, which, if left unattended, could be serious. Someone had to see to it that nothing was left in need of repair, and it seemed that I was now elected for the job.

Throughout the spring I made extra food for our suppers, packaging and labeling the extra portions for the freezer. I further prepared an index card with a list of the meals Jay could choose from. Our student friends had been alerted to visit him weekly, while our neighbors did whatever shopping he needed. Marie, who had been our general house helper, spent three mornings a week with him. All of this required considerable planning but it was worth the benefits: Jay realized that he was self-sufficient and that he had recovered from his stroke.

The years 1982 and 1983 were good for Jay. He filled them with the things he most liked to do: reading, listening to music, entertaining students and friends, and enjoying the leisure of retirement.

Since Jay's return from the Rusk Institute, I had undertaken his personal care. I became his hair-dresser and his manicurist for both hands and feet. It surely was a pleasant time, accompanied by much banter. I had a little library stool that moved on wheels until sitting on it clamped it to the floor. Liking the job, Jay's effusive enthusiasm for my work brought on one of my playful streaks. I finished his toenails and opened a bottle of red nail polish. "Whatever you do, don't put that on me," he yelled, pulling his feet back under his chair. I knew that this was precisely what he would say. Jay always prefaced his admonitions to me in the form of "*Whatever you do,* don't do. . . ." I pointed out to him that the way he put it implied that he believed that my possibilities for heinous conduct were unlimited, but it never sank in.

I waited awhile before I began again. Jay was particularly rigid about the way he wanted his hair cut. This time I conveniently forgot the mirrors. I had just finished the back of his head when he asked how it turned out. "Better than I expected," I replied.

Jay got suspicious. "Meaning *what*?" he asked.

"Well, I thought that the way you have been wearing it was a bit monotonous so I cut it into nicely even scallops." Jay rushed to the bathroom mirror to investigate the matter. I think he actually believed I might have done it.

On nice days we would drive to a pleasant and unfamiliar spot and enjoy a good walk. Jay walked slowly, painstakingly placing one foot ahead of the other. I found out not only how much more slowly he now walked but also how short I was on patience. I found it almost impossible to walk at this pace and would frequently find myself ahead of him, only to retrace my steps and return guiltily to his side. Neither my body nor my temperament seemed capable of being leisurely, but I made the excuse to myself that I was living an overly pressured life. I was attacking many tasks at top speed in order to get everything done. Even though my jobs included teaching courses, serving as chairperson of the department, doing the household shopping and cooking, paying the bills and keeping our financial records straight, and remaining in regular touch with our daughter, I felt guilty anyway.

In the summer of 1984, when I was assured that all was in readiness, I set off for the farm with my mind at ease. I was alone again since Jay, still remembering his anxiety, refused to accompany me. This time I left him in Marie's able "custodial care," which neither public nor private insurance paid for. (This was the first time that bills for Jay's care began to come in.)

The land was beautiful and the home inviting as I unloaded the car with enthusiasm. Then the phone rang with a nervous and worried Marie at the other end. Something had happened to Jay. He had suddenly become agitated and angry without any apparent cause. He was swearing, calling his visiting friends unpleasant names, and turning against her. No one seemed able to calm him, and I was asked to return home immediately.

I tried to be calm, pointing out that one had to expect unreasonable behavior from time to time because his brain had been scarred. I had seen a bit of this earlier when he would become sullen and uncommunicative for no apparent reason, but this time he seemed to have become actively combative. While I knew that brain damage was reversible, I also knew that stroke victims often harbored a corner of cussedness and recalcitrance, even when they had previously been gentle, affable, and good-hearted. I also knew that for a stroke victim unusual behavior could emerge from nowhere, at any time, and with no discernible cause.

I tried to calm Marie as well as visiting friends of Jay's, but one very close friend demanded that I return. I explained that it would all disappear as suddenly as it had come but she accused me of "selfishness" and neglecting my wifely duty. While I had seen Jay more or less like this before, this particular episode did seem out of bounds even for him. I speculated whether he might not have suddenly become aware of what he had been through and perhaps felt especially resentful, his anger being directed more at the fates than toward any particular person. And I wondered whether he might not be experiencing some dread regarding his future. However, I *am* sure that Jay, always the perfectionist in thought, diction, appearance, and action must have often experienced shame and embarrassment at his new insufficiencies and imperfections, which the stroke had produced. Still, I came home only to find everything at peace. This was the last rampage Jay ever had.

One night in March of 1984, I was in my study when, all of a sudden, there was a house-shaking crash from above. MY GOD! WHAT NOW? I bounded upstairs and there on the kitchen floor sat Jay, looking dazed. He was sitting flat on his behind with his legs stretched out in front of him, and he was leaning on his left elbow. What had he tripped over? I saw nothing, and all he would say was that he had "fallen."

The job now was to get him up. Only a gymnast could have stood up from that position. The rest of us would have needed to roll over on our side and get onto our knees. From the kneeling position we could more or less manage to return to our feet if there were something to hold on to. Being a small, light woman, I was no match for this tall, heavy-boned man. It didn't take me long to realize that I had to devise ways, albeit impromptu, of using anything and everything in sight, including my ingenuity, in order to handle the situation without help.

I selected a sturdy chair and brought it close enough so that Jay could put his hands on its seat. At this point I pushed him upward from the rear and quickly grabbed both of his hands. Our joint efforts finally resulted in Jay being pulled to his feet, after which I walked him slowly to his chair. He didn't know how he fell but I surmised (correctly, it turned out) that he had blacked out and dropped straight down. His view was that he fell and then became dazed by the fall. I reported this event to his doctor, and Jay was duly examined. The matter was called "an episode," which could be expected under the circumstances. I didn't really want to pursue the implications of "an episode." But subliminally I was aware that this had most probably been another ischemic attack. That awareness didn't help much at the time, because I had not yet heard of the carotid arteries. In retrospect, it is now clear to me that Jay's arteries needed the operation that could possibly have removed such wandering clots.

Typical of some ischemic attacks, their effects are neither quickly nor easily observed. The event seems to come and go without consequence. The trail of difficulties left behind usually occurs so gradually that its connection with the original cause is vague or even nonexistent. I found something especially damnable about this time lag between cause and effect in that it prevented me from seeing the whole picture and inhibited my ability to see, let alone prepare for, what might come next. Unable to discern recurrent patterns in the disease, I was set up to plunge headlong into yet another pitfall, namely, believing that Jay's increasing incapacity was not genuine but rather some sort of reluctance, rooted in fear and anxiety at best or obstinateness at worst. Like most people, I tended to believe that our actions are typically "voluntary," but when a stroke is involved, the difference between "I don't want to" and "I can't" is far from distinct. Perhaps this is because none of us want to admit the presence of a genuine disability that alters (in some cases permanently) tasks that we and the victims have performed all our lives. Furthermore, empathy with Jay led me to know very well about "not trusting oneself" with a task. So I cajoled and encouraged him to "try." I knew I should urge him to try, but it may well be that Jay couldn't even "try," much less "do." It almost seems that the dilemmas of those of us who nurture stroke patients are overly abundant. I think they are.

The only answer I could find to the problem was to keep both possibilities in mind. I would try a little cajoling and then give it up for awhile. I resolved to try it again and again. In this way it seemed possible to find out whether Jay's refusal to try a task stemmed from "I can't" or "I'm afraid to try."

At this point I found myself a hands-on caregiver and not just an overseer of the process. Engaging in hand-to-hand combat with the enemy caused me to see that the relation between the giver and the receiver of care is a kind of dance, a pas de deux, whereby each change in the receiver of care effects a reactive change in the giver. To encounter an "I can't" is an especially disturbing discovery, for the giver as well as the receiver of care. It reminded me of how deeply unnerved I was at the loud crash of Jay's fall; I had bounded up the stairs, shaking with apprehension and yelling. At the time, I felt guilty about this display of fear because I remembered one of the many unwritten rules of caregiving: the caregiver should always remain calm, loving, and patient. I think the "rule" requires reassessment. Armchair legislators of "proper" attitudes have never come to grips with emotional facts like the ones I was now facing with Jay. Emotions are readily communicated between people, all people, even strangers; but they are irrevocably communicated between people who are closely connected . . . sometimes as if there were no skin between them. If I'm anxious, Jay knows immediately: my body quivers, the tone of my voice changes, and my touch becomes urgent—almost frantic. It's no good trying to deny my feelings—that only increases Jay's fear. What really seems to help dispel the anxiety for both of us is just to begin helping in a business-like way, all the while explaining the trouble I may be having and asking for whatever help Jay feels capable of giving me. Although I may yet be shaking, Jay's attention is distracted by his own efforts to help and he is reassured by my actions.

Of course, there may be too much of anything, including empathy. I'm always a bit fearful that I'll lose my desire to aid; that I'll give in to giving up. If I start to fall apart in this way, I turn to less sensitized coworkers such as neighbors or the police.

Jay's fall caused his doctor to send us our first but not by any means our last "visiting nurse" to prepare a report on Jay's condition for his medical perusal. Our visitors were nuns connected with a Catholic parish and, I believed, were paid by Medicare—I know I never paid them. It seems that they give their lives to the service of visiting and treating the sick, helping and making suggestions to caregivers, and writing out very useful reports to doctors and hospitals regarding the patient's physical and psychological condition. All who visited Jay were, I believe, trained nurses by profession and inhabitants of a convent by conviction. Friendly, cheerful, gentle, and knowledgeable, they were both dedicated to their tasks and efficient in carrying them out. Not only did these visitors serve as useful intermediaries between our family and the medical establishment, but they personally performed many needed medical services. I was astonished by these contemporary nuns, who wore nurse's white uniforms, including those who substituted slacks for skirts, rather than a traditional clerical habit. Each and every one served as a pillar of strength and encouragement for me. While to them I was but a small part of their job—their calling—I have in fact been deeply grateful to them for their many kindnesses.

One day I began to notice something that I had probably observed before but had never really focused on: Jay's sensory responses had become hypersensitive. Any small sound, such as the ticking of a clock, seemed to him like a cannon blast, and he would ask that its source be removed. Patting him gently on the shoulder would produce not a smile but a pained "Ouch!" Coffee was always "too hot" and iced tea "too cold." His taste buds were over-alert, too: "Oh, that is *so* good!" or "Why did you make this *so* sour?" The visiting nurses told me that this was typical of stroke patients.

Although Jay had resumed his previous interests and preoccupations and seemed to be relatively normal, the doctor advised a follow-up CAT scan. This involved getting in and out of the car, which was no longer as easy for Jay as it had been. Again, I had to rely on ingenuity. I first learned to park the car at least a foot from the curb so that Jay could put both feet on the street before he took on the obstacle of the curb. Getting him out of the car required helping him use his legs in order to move sideways and face the open car door. From that vantage point he could grasp the top of the open door with his good left hand and, using the car frame for leverage with his right hand, he was able to stand upright. Only then did he need my hand to support him in his management of the curb. Getting into the car was the reverse process. First, he turned his back to the seat. Then, holding onto the door handle, he could let himself down onto the seat, sitting at a right angle to his final position. I would then help him get his legs into the car, at which point he would use his feet to turn himself around to face front. Standing beside him outside the car, I would lean over him to fasten his seat belt.

While waiting for the doctor's report on the scan, Jay and I nibbled at the picnic lunch I had prepared. Jay held a thermos cup for a moment and then promptly dropped it, spilling its contents all over himself. It was obvious that he was losing some of his "manual dexterity," and that made Jay all the more anxious, which in turn aggravated the problem. I made little of it but quietly took over holding the cup while he dealt with the sandwich. I noticed that he was chewing in an odd way, but I paid little attention to it.

The doctor's report, delivered privately to me, was that Jay's brain showed much additional scarring. The "fall" had injured more than just his dignity and pride.

Six months later, in October, as I worked on the monthly bills, there was another crash, and fear again ran through me as I discovered Jay, shocked and bewildered, sprawled out on the kitchen floor. He had duplicated his first "fall" at nearly the same spot in the kitchen. Again he sat on the floor, leaning on his left elbow. There was something eerie about this repetition of blackouts. They surely should have told me something, but I apparently didn't yet comprehend the message, again seeing each as an isolated event.

This time Jay found it much more difficult to regain his equilibrium. He became more and more fearful of walking and less inclined to try. I responded to the situation by hiring a young nurse to be with him all day. I brought out the cane that the Rusk Institute had made to order for him. This was not enough to steady his balance, so I brought out the claw-footed cane. But even this was inadequate, so we returned to the walker. In short, we were reversing the process by which he had recovered originally. Meantime, I started to rearrange his living conditions. The bathtub got a bath seat and hand grip. Instead of standing for his shower, he sat on the seat and used the hand shower we had formally used to bathe the dog. I had additional bannisters installed on all stairs (for the first time I realized that these helpful handrails are generally positioned for right-handed people). The nurse and I encouraged Jay to go up on the left side of the stairs and down on right rather than the customary procedure. His left hand was his only reliable balancing instrument.

Jay's motorized easy chair now came into serious use. Originally it had been purchased as a luxury to make him more comfortable, but now it became a necessity. It's seat rose mechanically to lift him onto his feet while he held onto its arms. It could return him to a sitting position by reversing the movements. Furthermore, when he wanted to nap, it would stretch him out by moving a headrest into position while a footrest moved out and up to support his legs in the lying-down position. In a few seconds he would be ready to nap without moving a muscle. All of this was done at the touch of a button. The chair was an oversized monster that dominated the living room but it was so helpful that I put aside my aesthetic concerns.

As Jay found it increasingly more difficult to walk and to climb the stairs to his second-floor bedroom, we both realized that he would have far less strain if he were to sleep on the first floor. It was then that I discovered what it meant for a house to be wonderously "versatile" in accommodating the needs of its occupants. We had chosen the plan for this home when we built it, but little did I know then how well we had chosen. Fortunately, the first floor had two bedrooms, one large and one small, with a complete bath to serve both. This choice made our living and dining rooms smaller, a decision over which I subsequently voiced regret because I like to entertain. Only a brief four years before Jay's first ischemic attack, I wanted to exchange the house for one more generous with entertaining space. Fortunately, I never found a satisfactory alternative. We were now able to house both Jay and Helen, the full-time live-in nurse, in comfortable and commodious surroundings. Had this not been a possibility, our struggle to cope with Jay's illness would have been compounded by moving to more suitable housing.

One morning I noticed that Jay's daily newspaper lay unopened on the floor. I watched for a week as it just sat there unread. Perhaps he needed new glasses. A visit to the opthalmologist was in order. Visits to doctors at this point were somewhat eye-catching to waiting-room occupants. I would face Jay, hold his hands, and walk backward while he would walk forward, feeling safe with this support. Together we maintained a brisk pace. Doctors, nurses, and waiting patients apparently understood the situation and smiled approvingly. I tended to play to the audience by producing some fancy steps which made Jay laugh.

The opthalmologist reported that Jay's *eyes* were in excellent condition and that his reading glasses were adequate. His was not a structural problem. Though Jay could read and understand the first sentence of whatever lay before him, he had forgotten what it said by the time he read the second sentence. In other words, Jay's ability to fund the meanings of a series of sentences had been lost. While he could understand and comprehend any *particular* sentence, he had lost the meaning connection when sentences were grouped in paragraphs. I stood silently as horror crept over me. *Jay had lost the power to read!* I never really came to grips with this forbidding result since it was a conclusion I couldn't fully absorb and one for which I had been entirely unprepared.

Nor had I ever known that this type of difficulty existed. It opened up a new kind of fear about the brain and its control over our abilities. Reading and writing had been central both to our individual lives and to our relationship. The Jay I had known for so long would never again be able to discuss, analyze, or criticize ideas. Gone now would be our vivid discussions as well as those he so often had with friends and students; these lively talks were his fondest pastimes. Gone would be his insights, his suggestions, and his penetrating comments that had so frequently and constructively sharpened my own understanding.

This could happen to me; it could happen to anyone! Putting myself in his place, I wondered what this new intellectual disfigurement felt like. Did he comprehend its implications? Did he understand what this meant for his very life-center; for the activities that he believed to be the source of his life's meaning and worth? I didn't dare to share these thoughts with Jay. Perhaps he was unaware of the overwhelming consequences of this new disability. Perhaps he could no longer see *any* picture as a whole.

I recalled my efforts to encourage Jay to write again after his retirement in 1982. Since he could no longer use his right hand, I thought he might be able to speak his thoughts onto a tape. So I modified his tape deck with a table-top microphone and a foot treadle that would stop the tape at will, giving him time to gather his next sentence together. He never used it. When I urged him to try, he commented, "Thoughts come from my head, across my feelings, and down my right arm to the pencil." And when I thought about it, that was the way it was with me, too.

As Jay's physical deterioration gradually but relentlessly continued, it was echoed by an equally gradual psychic transition from a fiercely independent person to a dependent one. Following suite without realizing it, my role imperceptibly moved from that of wife to caregiver; from second in command to the sole manager; from being "helped" to being a helper. I was responding to changes in Jay by taking on new roles without really being aware of them. My usual attention to what needed to be done, rather than on my attitudes toward it, caused me to slip into these new roles without noticing the contrasts between the present and the past.

Neither did Jay seem to notice his dependency on me. If he did, he didn't seem to resent it. I wondered whether his inability to play chess was an indication that he had lost some of connections between the memories of the past and the facts of the present. Perhaps the absence of complaint and resentment about his fate was due to some lack of time continuity in his thinking. If so, it was a blessing unnoticed by either of us.

I, on the other hand, continued to miss the conveniences with which he had previously provided me. Jay had always done the food shopping once a week, albeit with some grumbling. He explained his desire to perform this service on the grounds that I was an "impulse buyer," while he was more sensitive to the budget. But now shopping fell on my shoulders, and when time pressures were intense I often resented his contrasting ease in that big chair as I lugged in the bags.

Then, of course, there was the driving, which was now entirely my job. When our daughter visited and offered to drive, I expressed heartfelt gratitude for the privilege of sitting in the passenger seat. But my real sense of deprivation came when my car needed to be garaged for service. Previously, Jay would follow me in his car and drive me home, then bring me back to pick it up. In this new situation, I had to manage by either prevailing upon neighbors to perform his role or by selecting a garage near enough for a mechanic to drive me back.

Every night when the nurse had completed overseeing Jay's preparation for bed, I would come to sit with him, stroke his hair and kiss him. One night he quietly asked, "Will you lie with me?" The question was completely unexpected and a bit shocking; I was caught totally unprepared. I had never really thought about anything of this sort. But what sort was it? What did the question mean? I knew that long-time sexual mates tend to have a kind of subliminal awareness of each other as sexual partners. Jay's question would obviously have special overtones. I stumbled around looking for an answer. "Gosh!" was all I could muster. "Gosh!" I said again, having nothing further to contribute except, "You're on a hospital bed made for one, not two. I don't think it's a good idea." In short, I evaded coming to terms with his request, but I think about it to this day. Jay was asking a very serious question; he was looking to me for reassurance. Jay was asking, "Am I and my present physical condition as revolting to you as they are to me?" And in so many ways his psychic welfare depended on my answer.

This was precisely the issue that my father raised so many years ago. The memories started flooding my mind. He told me that my mother had asked him much the same question after her stroke. And in a voice filled with guilt and sorrow he told me that he could not comply, because the stroke had made her revolting to him. "Do you blame me?" he had asked, in a voice that told me he already blamed himself. Being only twenty-two at the time, I had not yet encountered the surds of this world.

The dilemma is sharp and intense. At first the caregiver is revolted at the ugly transformation of a beautiful and alluring mate into one distorted by a sick body and a failing head. Fear sets in. You just want to turn away and run. But then, overwhelmed by empathy, affection, and the vivid memories of previous sexual love and deep emotional connectedness, you reach out to comfort and heal the discomfort of your invalid spouse. I couldn't escape from the sword that hacked me into two irreconcilable parts. Had I been able to resolve this inner conflict, I would have contributed immensely to Jay's psychological and emotional well-being. Never again would I have been haunted by a failure to come to his aid in a time of psychological crisis. But that wasn't to be.

In another six months, almost to the day, Jay "fell" once more. Shortly thereafter, he seemed to have the same kind of chewing disorder I had noticed months earlier during our picnic. I decided to have his teeth checked. The dentist informed us that he had an infected wisdom tooth, which had to be removed. I dreaded the session with the dental surgeon. While Jay was having his tooth extracted, I relieved my anxiety by walking around the building. What a relief it was to see Jay emerge from the ordeal apparently intact. The tooth had been removed and the incision sutured. But what would he be like when the anesthesia wore off?

No sooner had we arrived home when Jay started to bleed profusely from the mouth. When the surgeon asked whether I was *sure* it was a hemorrhage, my emphatic *yes* brought on an immediate revisit. I stuffed a kitchen towel in his mouth, and this time his nurse came with us. More sutures were added and we again returned home. Jay was completely wilted after this ordeal. The nurse put him to bed, where he immediately fell asleep.

I dreaded the thought of Jay awakening, even though I had carefully put the codeine the dentist gave me within easy reach. Jay awoke. He was chipper and ready for his supper! I soon realized that Jay had never "come out" of the anesthesia, because he had been in it naturally all along! His mouth had been rendered numb by one of his "falls." *Now* I knew why his chewing at the picnic had been so odd, so clumsy. At the time it never occurred to me just how far this creeping paralysis might progress. The spacing of these episodic attacks and their results can be so distant that cause and effect relationships are often blurred or lost completely. This frustrating fact about stroke kept being driven home to me again and again over the years.

In looking back at the four years following Jay's retirement in 1982, I can see now how steep was his decline, which apparently stemmed from the minor "episodes" of falling. Cumulatively, they were not so "minor" even though individually they seemed to be relatively unimportant events in the broad scheme of things. Furthermore, this loss of ability was so gradual that I failed to realize its extent or its range. Time seemed to ease me into gradually getting used to small but continuous changes until suddenly, with shock and horror, I made the startling comparison between the "is" and the "was." I wondered how much Jay noticed and how he felt about the changes his mind and body were undergoing. Was he aware of a continuous decline? If so, he never complained about it, nor did he bemoan it. Rather, he noticed these limitations only when he could not do things that he had done previously. And when Jay did take notice of them, he did so only with a kind of silent resignation. When I asked him to read an article I had written, he said that he could only make comments on it concerning grammar and spelling errors! (Jay could read words but he could not comprehend the coherent connections between sentences, which add up to "meaning.") Even when it came to recognizing a loss of mental ability, he seemed simply to accept it!

I hesitated with great apprehension when it came to talking to Jay about his feeling toward capacities that seemed to deteriorate at an alarming rate. Perhaps he didn't notice them the way I did, even though I, too, took what was happening for granted. Only sudden memory flashes shocked me into perceiving how far my husband's condition had regressed and the extent to which his abilities had eroded.

The summer of 1985 again brought the time for my visit to Vermont to see to the welfare of our beloved mountain home. Thinking about what might best be done to assure Jay's well-being, I reviewed what I had done in previous years. In retrospect, this provided an eye-opening overview of the progress of his disease.

In 1982 it was possible to leave Jay alone in the house, since he was able to select and heat his own food, and the housekeeper would be able to check on him occasionally. That year I had prepared his food in the spring, frozen it, and provided him with an index of the menus. He was able to care for himself completely.

In 1983, I arranged for one of his graduate students to live in the house while she was completing her doctorate with him. This solution much relieved my mind, even though Jay was still capable of staying alone.

The whole of 1984 had been a quiet and good year for Jay as he listened to music and enjoyed the visits of his many student friends. Yet I instinctively felt that some check on him was needed. I persuaded our housekeeper-helper Marie to spend three mornings a week with him in order to see to his meals and keep him company.

Each of these summers I phoned Jay almost every night. I recall wanting to share with him a very humorous piano sonata for four hands by one of the Bach masters, which I had just taped from Maine Public Radio. I tried playing it into the telephone but with dubious results.

Jay had had two falls during 1985 and, as a result, his condition had considerably deteriorated. This time I asked Marie to "live in" during the week and supply me with a weekend helper since Jay now seemed to need closer attention.

In 1986, Jay fell two more times, each with its attendant consequences of lost abilities. Many physical problems had now developed for him and I was wary of leaving him at home with only one attendant. He had grown considerably weaker and I was concerned about another fall, since I knew that Marie could not bring him to his feet all by herself. Surveying the situation, I felt that Jay would be safer in a local nursing home as a temporary boarding patient until I returned. Should any further problem develop, I knew that it would be efficiently taken care of there. I didn't like this solution, but I felt more comfortable with it, despite the fact that I knew Jay probably wouldn't like it either. Yet, I was much too afraid of what *might* happen to entrust Jay to a single attendant without my help and supervision.

I acted on my convictions. I sought out a nursing home to board him for the time I would be away. While the administration of the facility flatly refused to accept Jay as a temporary resident, they changed their minds once they heard that he was a "self-paying patient" and that I was entirely willing to pay for the most expensive room in the house—which was, of course, "the only unoccupied room." The nursing home insisted on putting him in a wheelchair and binding him to it with a "restrainer," a new experience for him and for me—but of course so was the whole idea of a nursing home.

When I returned a few weeks later, Jay seemed none the worse for wear. I had dinner with him in his room and he not only ate all that he had been given but he handled the utensils reasonably well. I wheeled him to the elevator as I started for home. While waiting for the elevator to arrive, he looked at me so earnestly and said in a very quiet voice, "Will you take me home with you?" No words have ever etched themselves so deeply on whatever part of us it is that we call human. None had ever hit me more squarely in the heart. I assured him that I would take him home with me the next day.

The school year in the fall of 1987 began immediately to inflict its compounded pressures on my increasing difficulties at home. I was at the University five days a week. On the mornings of Monday, Wednesday, and Friday I taught three classes, each in an entirely different area of philosophy and each requiring separate preparation and teaching paraphernalia (e.g., samples, art reproductions, newspaper clippings, and assorted "show and tells"). These often had to be collected and organized the night before. In the afternoons, I tackled the department's mail and business, which consisted of everything from preparing its budget to proofreading pertinent sections of the college catalogue and answering requests for jobs, which, if we had any to fill, involved many meetings with the candidate, the department members, and the dean. Then, of course, there were the letters of recommendation for students who were seeking grants, entrance into graduate schools, and induction into honor societies. Faculty needed all sorts of letters and evaluations for increasing their salaries, reducing their teaching loads, and soliciting promotions. And there was, of course, the extensive paperwork required for getting new courses approved. Such operations required not only many departmental meetings but the leadership of the chairperson in formulating the needs, goals, and curriculum of the new course. Somewhere in the midst all of these activities I found time to eat a bag lunch since something more leisurely at the University Club was a luxury that one could only hope for.

Tuesdays and Thursdays were devoted to student conferences that ranged from going over their written work to discussions of personal, professional, and academic matters. In many ways, a teacher is a stand-in parent, a friend, and a confidante in students' eyes. Since I wanted to be comfortable, too, I made my office into a hospitable spot. It boasted a cabinet completely stocked with what I called, "broths for sick bodies and sick souls." A steaming electric kettle sat on top, ready to provide everything from herbal teas, coffee, and hot chocolate to packaged soup and snacks for the hungry whose pocket money had run out.

Tuesdays and Thursdays brought a plethora of meetings of which a University hatches an extensive brood. All too frequently, chairpersons were expected to be on board. These, too, had their out-of-meeting demands since they were often advisory to various levels of administrators. Reports and well-thought-out recommendations were expected.

On the way home I would shop for everything from groceries to hardware to "sundries" for all concerned. Then I would rush home to cook dinner, sometimes with hat and scarf still on, until Nurse Helen would giggle at the sight.

All three of us enjoyed our dinner together. (It couldn't have been made, of course, unless it had been planned in transit.) I enjoyed simply not having to think; Jay enjoyed his food, as he always had; and Nurse Helen enjoyed becoming friend and half-family with us. Helen would talk of Jay's day, and I would tell both of them about mine. Jay would join in once in a while.

After Helen tidied the kitchen, and we all reviewed a bit of the national and international news of the day, she would ready Jay for bed. I would spend a few minutes of quiet time with him, then I'd rush off to my disordered study. Books were all over the floor by my chair; notes about calls to be made were scattered around the phone; mail was all over the desk; and notes were hanging helter-skelter from a very large bulletin board, which I typically avoided since it reminded me of things I should have done last week but didn't.

The real question of each evening was, of course, what to do first. I tried to avoid lingering over that question lest *nothing* would be accomplished. Should I open last week's mail? Should I spend the evening opening the mail for both weeks and pay the bills lurking in the large pile of "junk mail" and requests for money in behalf of "causes"? On second thought, that move would bring me face to face with the fact that I hadn't balanced either Jay's checkbook or mine. How could I enter new checks with that operation still undone?

The telephone rang. A colleague wanted to know whether I had the reference he asked me to look up for him. (Good heavens, I had forgotten that.) I went back to the desk, and this caused me to remember that I had to prepare for my classes the next day. (Good grief, I also had to round up the illustrations I needed for the arts class.)

The phone rang again. It was our daughter wanting to talk out a problem she was facing. Of course I gave the time, but I was looking anxiously at the clock. We worked it out and I returned to the desk. Then Helen appeared at the door.

"I forgot to tell you that the dryer stopped cold in the middle of a load today."

"I'll put it in my daybook to call the repairman tomorrow. *Where is* that daybook? I ought to get it in there before I forget. And *that* reminds me, I forgot to tell the Vermont plumber that the house needs winterizing. *Where* is that daybook?" (I had often declared that, were it lost, I would have to be reincarnated and start again from scratch.) Once it *was* lost in the summer. Really lost. I returned to New York and found in the mail a notice to the effect that because I had not paid my taxes, our New York home was to be put on the auction block! Jay's comment on my financial ineptitude that "time will wait; you will slowly drift into satisfaction" now needed amending. I didn't wait and I dashed into vituperation. A fiery letter to the tax officials pointing out that I had never received the notice brought an eventual apology.

Returning again to the desk, I absent-mindedly opened the first letter. It announced "This bill is OVERDUE!" Not wanting to awaken Jay with a bloodcurdling scream of frustration, I muttered under my breath, "It is *not* and I can prove it," that is if the weekend I devote to unscrambling all of this is long enough to make some headway. But in my annoyance I pushed the pile of mail, and what would come into view but the daybook. It was midnight and I suddenly realized that I was suffering the lethal combination of being both exhausted and frustrated. What really had gotten done?

Jay's days could not have been in greater contrast to mine. Having slept twelve hours, he was awakened at nine A.M. by the cheerful, melodious voice of Nurse Helen. He was leisurely washed, dressed, and helped into the wheelchair for breakfast. Then he was moved to his lift-chair, made comfortable with a sweater and a blanket in order to spend the rest of the morning listening to his favorite classical music station and/or the daily news. The radio receiver was set to permit alteration between these two with a touch of a button.

Lunch followed at one in the afternoon, after which Helen would help him back to bed for a nap of an hour or two. Weather permitting, the restful sleep would be followed by some fresh air. Helen would carefully help Jay down the stairs and into his wheelchair for a brief jaunt around the neighborhood. She would then return him to bed for a nap before supper. Jay's perpetual exhaustion seemed to warrant putting him to bed at nine P.M. At this point he was sleeping fifteen or sixteen hours a day. He had a regularized, totally predictable life of complete monotony. Yet he seemed content with it. He wasn't restless, nor did he complain. I measured his deterioration by his docility and agreeable acceptance of this regime. He couldn't read, write, take walks, or even play a game of checkers. He couldn't use his hands for crafts. Nor could I take him for rides in the car, because it was both difficult to get him in and out of the car and he retained his phobic response to sitting in the passenger seat.

I am not sure whether it was the extreme contrast between our lives or just that good sense had finally overtaken me in my frenetic activity, but, for a change, I took stock of the impossible burden I carried. While I had always been known for having an overabundance of energy, I began noticing not only that I was running out of steam, but that I was becoming increasingly more irritable each time I faced the chores awaiting me in the "study." (Who was studying? Who was writing the articles I wanted to write?) It was already four years since I had written an intensely serious piece on "Ethics and the Environment," and three years since I was asked to celebrate the addition of the millionth volume to our University library by delivering a speech on "My Creative Experience in Writing a Book." The latter was a humorous presentation with "creative experience" being in quotes. I missed this type of effort. Meantime, I had been told that Jay's deterioration was such that I was in for a long, hard pull.

Within the space of one evening I radically changed my long academic life. First, I decided to resign the chairmanship within two months, at the end of the fall semester 1986. Second, that the year 1988 to 1989 would be my last year of teaching and that I would retire at the end of the spring semester 1989. This would coincide with my fortieth year at the University. Third, that my last year would be spent teaching half-time; I would rely on my pension to provide the other half, thus maintaining my income at its present level. I would then be prepared to face Jay's subsequent bouts with stroke.

5

The Second Knock-Down Blow (1987)

New Year's Eve 1986 saw me keeping vigil with Helen. As we watched the merrymakers across the country, I wondered why they should be so happy about the coming of the New Year. How could they know that it wouldn't bring sorrow and mishap? Could they have such faith in the beneficence of the universe as to believe that it would bring only joy and fulfillment? I remembered Jay once saying that it wasn't a "celebration" at all but a kind of mass hysteria that hid doubt, fear, and foreboding; a kind of together-shouting to drown out doubt and apprehension. Helen and I were both quiet. I suggested that we enter into the spirit of the moment with a good-night drink.

When the first day of the new year brought the sun, Helen told me that something strange seemed to have happened to Jay. When she went to bathe, change, and dress him, he refused to open his eyes. Previously he would stare at her, indicate recognition with a grunt, and help her as best he could with the arduous tasks of preparing him for a day in his big chair, listening to the news and to his much loved classical music. But this day, no matter how lively and cheerful she was, Jay ignored her, lost, I thought, in some sort of recalcitrance— or was it torpidity? Something had indeed happened, but what? What were we to expect now?

We left Jay in bed for the day since he showed no inclination to come alive. The buttons to his hospital bed were used to command him into awakening by raising him into a sitting position, but his eyes would open sleepily for a second and then close again. With his head lolling sideways on his neck, Jay shut out the world—or was it being shut out for him? He wouldn't open his mouth for food to be spooned in, an unusual event for him since he typically cooperated eagerly in this procedure.

After a few days of near total inertia, Jay began to return to life, more or less. It was at this point that we began to see how this last brain-event manifested itself: first on the limpness of his legs, and second on his slurred speech. Jay's efforts to stand were hesitant, and his gait—when he tried, that is—was weak and wobbily, requiring far more assistance than just a steady arm to hold. Now one of us had to put one arm completely around his waist. His efforts to walk were so painful to watch that, whenever possible, we eased him into the wheelchair. I was encouraged that he could still obey the command to lift his feet and place them on the wheelchair footrests. He seemed too exhausted and weak to stay awake and often lapsed into sleep.

We tried to keep his interest in music alive and to engage his comments regarding the news of the day. He listened and tried to comment, but his speech was so distorted that I had difficulty understanding what he said. "Would you say that again?" I'd ask, and then I would listen intently. Eventually I would understand him, but the effort for both of us was exhausting. Jay understood. He began to answer using just yes and no; he said "Ah!" in approval, while he ugged in disapproval and grunted to indicate his understanding of what was being said. He communciated, but he was reluctant to verbalize.

While there can be, and often is, nonverbal communication between humans, much as there is in the animal world, humans naturally accept structured language as their primary form of interaction. Without words serving as an exchange between separate selves, each is more or less "alone" in a special kind of way. I was encountering just how frustrated and perplexed humans could be without verbal exchange. My grief at this diminished capacity in Jay was the deepest I have ever known. It reminded me of one version of the wonderful Greek tale of the lovers Orpheus and Eurydice. Eurydice died prematurely, and Orpheus grieved so severely that even Zeus, the Greek god of gods, was unnerved. Zeus finally gave Orpheus the right to journey to the Underworld to be with Eurydice on the single condition that he did not speak to her. Should he do so, he would never see her again. Orpheus arrived in the Underworld, and there was Eurydice who immediately reached out to him with many words of love. Orpheus remained silent, as he had been commanded. Eurydice pleaded for Orpheus to speak to her. Then she intensified her demand by asking whether he loved her. Did he *really* love her? If he did, he would speak and say so. As she pleaded, Orpheus was psychologically pushed to the wall both by the question and her insistence. Overwhelmed by love and unable to help himself, he responded. As Zeus had decreed, Orpheus immediately disappeared from her sight. At this point Eurydice took her turn at loudly proclaiming *her* bereavement after her short-lived happiness. She grieved so intensely that Zeus saw his error. He really couldn't reduce human beings to wordless animals. He was asking too much and he knew it. Concluding, apparently, that human beings *had* to have verbal communication in order to live as nature intended, he revoked the order and permanently reunited the lovers. Where was my Zeus when I needed him!

Helen and I had already concluded, almost immediately, that Jay had indeed experienced another "cerebral episode" on New Year's Eve, and we were soon to have more evidence of it. Jay now seemed to have to make overly frequent trips to the bathroom, and getting there was becoming increasingly more difficult. Had his prostate, which had previously been operated on, become bothersome again? When, once too often, he suffered the embarrassment of not making the journey in time, we decided to try making things easier for him (and, yes, for us) by putting him into disposable diapers made of plastic and padding over which we put waterproof underpants similar to those used on a baby. This move was also accompanied by putting a small disposable waterproof mat across the middle of his bed. Both diapers and mats come in large quantities housed in mammoth cartons that the druggist was delighted to deliver since considerable profit can be made on such items. But there was a down side to these efforts designed to increase Jay's comfort and his peace of mind. The plastic made the garments airtight; Jay's skin couldn't "breathe." In young children this typically results in a bad case of "diaper rash," which can be remedied by removing the waterproofing for a while and treating the area with powders, salves, and lotions. Unlike active infants, a stroke patient is basically motionless; here the result is not merely diaper rash but bedsores or "decubitae."

When I first heard about bedsores I believed them to be only a fancy name for the "garden variety" of sore. I also believed that I could heal any type of sore with an appropriate ointment. So what's a bedsore and why should everyone speak of them with so much dread? (Most of my fantasies about home care of the stroke victim were overly optimistic, complete with ignorance of the facts.) I soon found out.

A bedsore is a pressure ulcer that first appears as a red irritation on certain sections of the skin where the pressure of the patient's weight has been too insistently present. In Jay's case these irritations occurred on the sides of both hips where the pressure of sitting was compounded by the pressure of lying on these same areas, which were under constant pressure both day and night. While a decubita begins as a red rash, the area soon deteriorates to a point at which the skin breaks open and "weeps." The weeping develops into a crust or a scab, which, in Jay's case, was first white in color but then turned black. Meanwhile, under the scab, the micro-organisms that cause the sores begin to imperceptibly destroy more and more healthy tissue. These ulcers are actually a form of gangrene, and once having gained a foothold there is no easy reprieve. In many cases where poor circulation results from inactivity, bedsores on heels and legs can force physicians to amputate. But a hip can't be amputated: the sores resist healing regardless of lotions, antiseptics, or ointments. As time goes on, they not only deepen but enlarge.

We positioned pieces of "fleece cloth" around the affected areas to try to lessen the pressure on them, but to no avail. I made urgent pleas to the doctor for antibiotic ointment—anything that might stop the progress of Jay's sores—but the prevailing medical opinion was deeply discouraging. Any antibiotic that would kill the organisms causing these sores would also kill the patient. Any antiseptic strong enough to be effective would result in skin burns that would not heal. It was apparent that I couldn't win over these devils—at least not in any ordinary way. We kept trying nonetheless. Morning and night saw bouts of washing, treating, and bandaging these lesions; devotedly we turned Jay regularly from side to side, but since he had a sore on either side, the effort amounted to very little.

The only mitigating feature of decubitae is that in the process of turning healthy tissue into infected pulp, they mercifully kill the nerve endings in the affected areas. While they are both revolting and life-threatening, they don't hurt as much as their appearance would suggest. The experience of pain is one of the major vehicles the body has to assist us in gauging when medical attention is needed and when treatment is working. Without this natural barometer, it was difficult to tell when we were helping Jay and when we were injuring him.

Jay's doctor again appealed to Medicare to pay for visiting nurses who would report to him regarding the state of our battle with this microscopic enemy. Medicare concurred and we were given an allowance of a number of visits by these delightful and efficient emissaries of mercy. The reports were all pessimistic. I couldn't believe that, despite our efforts, we were losing the battle. While I could see that the lesions had appropriated more territory, there was no way to tell what was happening below the scab. For this reason I wasn't inclined to believe the nurses' reports.

Throughout the long process of Jay's ailment, I had taken note of the deficiencies of our home with regard to caring for his increasing disability. Now I took another look and set about remedying those obstacles I had not overcome earlier. First, the bathroom door was too narrow for Jay's wheelchair. We had to leave the chair at the door and then help Jay to the toilet or the tub. I got an estimate on the cost of widening the door but decided to wait until this was absolutely necessary. Second, the old wooden thresholds at the bottom of the doorways were a drawback for the wheelchair attendant, so we removed all of them. Third, I had not previously anticipated the need for a railing that Jay could hold on to while he was being dressed. The towel bar often served as a handy substitute. However, one day it pulled out of the wall and he fell backward onto the nurse and both landed on the bathroom floor. Neither was hurt but both were well shaken. It did provide a good laugh for all when the shaking subsided. I had a new bar installed, but even though it was steel and anchored in the studs of the house rather than in the wall, Jay never quite overcame his doubts about its stability. Fourth, the toilet was positioned too low, not only for Jay but for anyone who is tall or who has arthritis, back injuries, or muscle problems. The problem was resolved when I heard about and subsequently purchased a lightweight styrofoam "seat raiser" that elevated the seat six to eight inches. Just that small adjustment made getting on and off the toilet remarkably easy. (How I wish I had known about it when I spent three months recovering from a broken rib.)

Even ordinary table utensils failed to be adequate. Stroke victims need a plate that anchors to the table with suction cups so that it doesn't "walk away." Here the Rusk Institute had supplied the answer when it sent Jay home with a plastic plate equipped with suction cups on the bottom. It was also divided into sections with raised sides in order to hold the food in as he pushed it to the side. The food stayed on the plate so he could then get it onto a spoon or fork. The Institute also sent an ingenious eating utensil, a fork with serrated edges for cutting. All of this was designed with one-handed eating in mind.

The Rusk Institute had also supplied Jay with a clipboard to hold writing paper steady and a thick-handled pencil that he was able to hold on to. Since his was a stroke affecting the right side, Jay was obliged to learn how to write left-handed. Rusk therapists had started him on this practice but Jay had such great difficulty shifting from his lifelong right-handedness that soon he gave up all efforts in this direction. Meantime, the hospital bed and motorized easy chair, which had been great conveniences at first, now became absolute necessities. It was a great comfort to know that Medicare typically pays for these.

One morning Helen called me. Jay was on the floor beside the bathroom sink and she was unable to bring him back to his feet. I rushed in and took one arm while she grabbed the other. With considerable effort we brought Jay to his feet. He steadied himself by holding on to the sink. A second later, as our grasp on him loosened, he crumpled again to the floor. Once more we struggled and succeeded in getting him up, only this time we held on while maneuvering him into the wheelchair, which we had positioned to receive him. I wondered what I would have or could have done alone in such a situation. Jay's legs seemed to have turned to putty. I was so grateful that the nurse was with me.

New facts, which this latest episode revealed, began to dawn on me. Jay was having serious trouble standing up, even with help on either side. His inability to support his own body with his legs brought on an altogether new way of life for all of us. For one thing, it was difficult if not impossible to dress him. This was not only a problem in itself but a serious blow to Jay's self-image. Instead of clothes, he now had to be wrapped from waist to feet in blankets. Shirts and sweaters were more difficult to put on than one would imagine, both because of his inability to help and because his back was always leaning against something. While a patient in this condition may not be bedridden, the new situation removed his sense of dignity and well-being once and for all. Furthermore, and perhaps more importantly, Jay's new situation meant that he couldn't help himself move anywhere, whether it be getting in and out of bed or transferring from the bed to the wheelchair or from the wheelchair to the motorized easy chair. In each case he virtually had to be carried.

These new facts brought about a third consideration: Jay could no longer be cared for by female nurses (unless it was possible to afford two) because they are not physically strong enough to manage such negotiations with a tall, bony man. The time had now come to bring in two strong, efficient male nurses: one for weekdays and nights and one for the weekend days and nights.

This was far easier to contemplate than to accomplish. Male nurses are scarce at the best of times, and those who are available are frequently snapped up by eager hospitals. I called several agencies but was told that they had not had such applicants for several years. Desperation brought to mind the possibility of nursing home placement. Though I hated the thought of Jay being institutionalized, I decided that I had to consider the prospect.

Making a list of a dozen homes in the vicinity, I made a pilgrimage to each, carrying with me the calling card for which they all asked, namely, the overview of Jay's total condition, which had been so neatly and efficiently prepared by the visiting nurses. Several homes told me that they had a waiting list and that it could be a year or more before a vacancy would develop. Others told me that they didn't have enough skilled nurses on staff to care for Jay's needs. One home frankly told me that he was "too sick" to be admitted. What did "too sick" mean? Did it mean that they only wanted to admit those who required little care? Did it mean that if he were *that* sick, it was time to die and get it over with? Indeed, there was "no room at the inn"! I returned from these visits with a sense of utter helplessness and desolation. It was up to me to resolve this impasse. But how? All roads were blocked!

My face began to itch and then burn with scratching. A quick glance in the mirror revealed that my face was covered with large, bright red splotches. I should have expected this: just a few days earlier my tongue had been sore, my ears itched and "ran," and my nose had been running. Of all times to plague me, why now? It was, of course, my lifelong barometer, infallibly and accurately measuring the level of my internal stress. It was eczema, which I had been told could take on dozens of forms, depending on the location where it takes up habitation in order to raucously announce that an emotional breaking point is close at hand. In this case it emerged *everywhere*. A bathtub of high-powered cortesone could not have been enough to bring these dermatological red flags down. The only way to move on such an internal explosion was to try to solve the problem that caused the outbreak in the first place.

I decided to try new agencies this time. I knew that male attendants were scarce but I refused to believe that they were extinct. I was already aware that they preferred the eight-hour hospital day to the twenty-four-hour one that was expected in home care.

Panic set in. Panic, for me, often starts a flow of improbable and sometimes outrageous solutions. After all, Jay didn't need "nursing" care. He needed extensive custodial care from a man with well-developed muscles. With this in mind I thought that perhaps I could roam the hospital corridors until I saw a white-clad male washing the floors. I would then engage him in light conversation, starting with the detergent he was using. I would then praise his excellent work and offer some comments about good versus bad floor washing, etc. After friendly rapport was established, I would offer him a cigarette, which would automatically take us outdoors and onto neutral ground. At this point I would "pop" the leading question: "How much do you get paid for this menial job?" This would be followed by "How would you like to have one that would pay double and that comes with your own room, television, air conditioner, and time to nap in the afternoon when your charge does?"

I didn't really want to stoop to this pirating, at least not yet. I put plotting aside to try the normal route again. This time I called an agency that I had previously used for other types of help. I didn't believe what I heard; surely I was mistaken! The owner had told me that the first male nursing attendant they had seen in months was sitting there now, filling out papers! Chuck was hired on the spot, sight unseen! What unbelievable luck! As relief washed over me I was again reminded of my isolated and lonely childhood, equipped with its fertile imagination. I had believed that not only "folks" visited me but that I had a guardian angel who came when I was in trouble and had nowhere to turn. I think that I again heard her wings flap as she took off, having accomplished her mission!

Chuck was a young black man, small, wiry, and extremely strong. Pleasant, cheerful, and cooperative, he was a joy to have around the house, and it wasn't long before he became a rock on which I could rely. He had wanted to be a physician, but money and circumstances had thwarted this intention. He came complete with a cheap stethoscope, a still cheaper blood-pressure machine, and a thermometer. It was obvious that he deeply wanted a medical career, and I regretted that our society was not prepared to give what seemed to be incipient talent a chance to get the necessary education. In any case, he made an excellent male nurse.

As it turned out, Chuck had a friend who could take over on the weekends, provided he could sleep several hours after he arrived on Saturday mornings because he played in a band on Friday nights! Considering my need, anything was acceptable. Bill, the band player, raised his stock by exhibiting his strength to me. He picked up Jay as one would a baby and carried him into the kitchen. At least this special asset compensated for an unusual liability. It was good to know that Jay would never again lie helplessly on the floor waiting for aid from some unknown source. Things were looking up, I felt.

However, I began to realize just how fragile were the ties that held my household together and with what weak strings it was maintained intact. Without a nursing home to turn to in a pinch and with the nursing help I had recently hired—a freak accident at best—I was in a precarious position despite appearances.

I also began to see the bills for Jay's illness rise precipitously. The male attendants were more expensive than the female ones, starting at a hundred dollars a day and moving upward apace. The grocery bills began to triple because the men were hungry. The "supplies" (bandages, antiseptics, diapers, bed pads, nurses gloves, medicine, etc.) all proceeded to sap what there was of Jay's fairly good pension and Social Security checks. I was still working and making a good salary, but it had to stretch to maintain both me and our two homes. I was beginning to feel the pinch. Medicare didn't pay either for the "custodial care" we had had for four years or for the more serious, round-the-clock home nursing we had had for the last two years. Medicare, however, did pay for "special" nursing care for a few hours a day for a certain allowable number of days. But Jay needed continuous care day and night, seven days a week. My thoughts and my heart went out to my fellow caregivers who either were not or could not be eligible for Medicaid but whose incomes were not large enough to take on full-time nursing care. I was lucky. Our combined incomes could do it. The question was, for how long, especially with the cost of care continuing to increase.

6

The Knockout Blow (1988)

It was early March 1988 and I decided to take a day or two off to attend a conference of colleagues meeting at State College in Pennsylvania. Many of my old friends would be there. Because of my many obligations at home, I hadn't seen them for a long time and was eager to make their reacquaintance. Things were going well with Jay, and Chuck was not only an excellent nurse but his cheerfulness was a pleasure to have around. A good friend and I started on the beautiful drive through the Alleghenies about noon on a Thursday. It snowed lightly as we drove through the mountains. Finally, I felt myself relaxing. The site of this meeting was a charming old hotel complete with chamber music in the lobby. For the first time in many months I felt in a holiday mood. What a treat it would be just to sit down and listen to academic papers for a change.

While we sat at dinner one of Jay's most devoted students came running in my direction. "*At last* you're here" she fairly shouted, "because I don't know what has happened!"

"What has?" I asked, a bit taken back at her obvious distress. It seems that she had called our home before boarding the plane in New York. No one answered! She tried again in Pittsburgh and the same thing happened. Upon arriving at the conference she tried again, with the same result.

As I tried to digest this unwelcome news, I felt consternation grasping at my throat. We tried to call from my room but still no answer. Every imaginable horror passed thrugh my mind. Had Chuck fallen down the cellar stairs and broken a leg or received a blow to the head rendering him unconscious? Where was Jay? Had he suddenly become ill and had Chuck gone with him to a hospital? What now? Who had a house key? How would I tend by long distance to whatever went wrong?

My first thought was to call a friend who had a key. No one answered! I then called my next door neighbor and asked him to walk around the house and look in the windows to see what he could. Sweat was trickling down my back, and my legs felt weak. I sat on the bed as anxiety and trembling set in. What *had* happened?

The telephone rang. It was my neighbor reporting that the lights were on and that Jay was sitting in his motorized chair, shaking his fist! There had been no sign of Chuck.

All that I could muster by way of solution was "Oh my God, my God, my God!" I could feel that the problem, whatever it was, was urgent, but I didn't know what to do next. I did know that Jay was either about to have or already had another serious stroke. His days had been so uneventful and regularized that anything so unusual would be a shock. Besides, he was too incapacitated to handle an event that would, under the best of circumstances, totally disorder him. He was shaking a clenched fist and I was already too familiar with the effects of anger on him.

My mind sorted through the names of everyone I could conceivably contact and it feverishly landed on Marie, who had earlier taken care of him and still had her key. It was getting late but I had to take the chance. Marie answered sleepily, but she quickly became wide awake at hearing of my plight and its mystery. She and her husband would dress and go immediately. Even though help was on the way, my fear continued unabated. I spent the longest hour of my life waiting for her report.

Marie called back to say that she didn't need the key, because the back door was open! Chuck was nowhere to be found. She gathered that Jay had been sitting in his chair for about twelve hours without food, water, or diapering! Marie and her husband set about taking care of Jay's needs, putting him to bed, and then waiting. Chuck returned at three in the morning! What in the name of heaven had happened?

I stayed in my motel room to see if I could find out. It wasn't long before Chuck called. His mother had called him to say that his sister, who was battling cancer, had been taken to the hospital and she needed him to help her deal with the situation. But it wasn't long after hanging up the phone with Chuck that Marie called to say that his whole story was a lie. I then called Chuck's mother, who also denied the whole story but she added that the problem was with Chuck's uncle, "a bad influence" on him, who must have urged Chuck "to go out carousing."

What was this all about? Had Chuck been drunk or on drugs? How *could* he have left Jay helpless and unattended? I was both angry and confused. This was entirely unlike the Chuck I had known for nearly a year.

Then Chuck called again, contrite, and the uncle also called to apologize. At this point I trusted nothing. A few hours later I called the house only to find a cheerful Chuck on the job reporting that Jay was fine and eating well. I didn't believe it!

I hadn't been to a single meeting and I hadn't met a single friend. I wasn't to do so on this trip. I hadn't solved the mystery and could think about nothing else until I did. Maybe I dreamed this whole thing! I began to feel ill and wanted to do nothing more than get back home in a hurry. But I took another shot at solving this conundrum and called Chuck's mother again. Recognizing my voice, she began to cry.

"I don't understand his behavior," I told her, "he seems to be two entirely different people!"

"It's odd that you say that," she responded, "since you are the second one who has said this."

"Who was the first?" I asked.

"The first was his wife, who divorced him for that reason."

Suddenly it dawned on me! Chuck had a classic case of schizophrenia! The Chuck who had so gently and respectfully tended Jay, and the Chuck who so cruelly abandoned him, simply didn't know one another, except vaguely and unclearly.

When I returned home, Jay was sitting in his chair: his favorite music was on and he had been washed, dressed, and fed. Chuck, who was tending to business with the ever-present laundry, greeted me warmly and amiably with his usual good humor. As usual, my response to Chuck's misdeed was outwardly calm. I had liked and depended on him so much that I deeply regretted having to let him go. Besides, how could I be angry when I knew that he had serious psychological problems? Both he and I knew that a rigid rule of nursing, much like that of "the changing of the guard," is that a nurse may *never* leave a patient until a replacement arrives. But I was in no hurry to bring on immediate termination since the problem of replacing Chuck loomed overhead. I couldn't help feeling that this must have been just a very bad dream. I never expected to have so many problems with home nursing.

Marie, who always seemed to come to my aid, asked me to interview a neighbor from "her" island in the Caribbean. He had just arrived in this country. "Her" island always seemed to me to consist of a large, extended family. Her neighbor Joe had nursed before and he needed a job. I hired him sight unseen!

Joe was a small but very athletic young black man who turned out to be an artist, painting rather moving pictures of native life on "the" island. He displayed them for me eagerly. There was a group catching fish in a net, community style; children dancing; native musicians on a broken-down porch, playing homemade instruments; and some arresting samples of the native scenery. One of Joe's pictures was in the British Embassy there, he told me with great pride. He spoke the king's English with a slightly British accent. Wonders never cease, I thought.

Up to that point I had not had the time to notice changes in Jay. I don't think I wanted to look. My duties at the University were so incredibly demanding that I was content to let stand whatever seemed to be going well without further scrutiny. Of course, Jay had another stroke. I knew it but I didn't want to become fully conscious of it lest it be more severe than the last one. It was.

The first thing I let myself notice was that Jay had another bout with the desire to sleep. I protested to Joe and asked him to keep Jay awake during the day. Joe responded that he had tried to do just that but to no avail.

"He just falls asleep in his chair, and if he needs to sleep that badly, it is best that he be able to stretch out on his bed," Joe said.

The next thing I noticed was that Jay seemed to get tired trying to reach his mouth when eating. He simply didn't seem to be able to find his mouth with his hand, sometimes hitting his chin with the spoon and at other times hitting his cheek. Then he would put the spoon down and give up. Joe took over and began to feed him. When this happened, Jay continued to eat. Joe fed Jay from that point on.

Then one morning, purely by accident, I looked in on Jay and I saw Joe grab him under his arms and swing him from the side of the bed onto the wheelchair. "Why don't you help him try to stand first and then help him into the chair?" I asked.

"Because he *can't* stand up," Joe answered.

I seemed to have forgotten that he couldn't. Did I really want so much to believe he would "get over it" that I couldn't face the facts I already knew? Meanwhile, Jay stared ahead blankly during this conversation. This was surely worse than anything I had seen to date. Jay had not responded to the conversation in any way. Then I wondered whether he did or did not understand what was said. How could I tell if there was absolutely no response, not even a subtle if silent mouth movement or a head nod or a lifted eyebrow or a grunt? And even if any of these had occurred, would I be "reading in" a nonexistent understanding?

When communication totally fails or is given up, caregivers enter a new role. They have to deal with total lack of input. Therefore, any and all decisions made *for* the victim become problematic. When "Are you cold?" or "Are you uncomfortable?" meet with no reassuring response, how does one know what the better thing to do is?

September 1988 brought new events closely related to Jay's March trauma, which had not yet worked its way out of him. Much as Jay seemed to enjoy his food, sooner or later, *eating* produced a choking seizure. I became both nervous and impatient with these all too frequent episodes of unpredictable choking; they made our dinners both unpleasant and apprehensive, not at all conducive to the conviviality that dinners together should have. Of course, I fell into one of the typical pitfalls. I scolded Jay and admonished him to eat more carefully. I asked Joe to feed him smaller spoonfuls and to wait until Jay had swallowed before giving him more. Again, I was assuming that all of this could be avoided, if only greater care were taken.

One evening when I was at my desk, up to my elbows in bills, filing, financial matters, unresolved household problems, and a flood of medical paperwork, all of which had to be done before preparing for my next day's classes, Joe appeared. Jay was coughing, breathing heavily, and had a fever of 103! Naturally, the first move would be to "call the doctor," but no doctor ever makes housecalls. Either they were not in their offices, leaving only the answering service to respond with "The doctor will call you back . . . ," or no one would answer. Today, doctors so routinely rely on the machinery surrounding them in both offices and hospitals that they can't really practice without it. I had previously recognized Jay's need for a monthly check-up but this involved getting him either to a doctor's office or a hospital (which most doctors preferred, because a hospital provides not only a battery of machinery but an on-the-spot lab as well).

To deal with the special problem of home medical care for a bed-ridden patient, I had tried to enroll Jay as a member of the hospital's new Geriatric Center, where a "member" was assured of a monthly doctor's visit. I applied, was interviewed at length, and then denied admittance. I wrote a letter of appeal and requested that they reconsider the decision. It wasn't answered. I finally secured another appointment. In the waiting room, I took note of the members of this geriatric enclave. They were all, without exception, in their early sixties, mobile, and alert. I could come to no other conclusion than that Jay was denied admittance due to his being too far gone—too sick, too old (seventy-four), and too helpless. In short, those who most needed this help were denied it.

Joe's announcement brought me to Jay's bedside. He was obviously very ill, and this time it was not with the stroke per se. This conclusion successfully avoided one of the most persistent pitfalls in tending a stroke patient—the conviction that all illness is an effect of stroke. Now, in the long run, it typically is. Yet attention can be so riveted on stroke and its aftermath that it is difficult to see other troubles. After all, sleepiness could be caused by physical troubles other than stroke. But the nurse seems caught in "L'idea fixe." He thinks stroke first, if for no other reason than that this ailment typically tends to display new and unfamiliar symptoms. He thinks and sees with stroke-filled eyes; it is difficult to switch into another gear and think of other possibilities.

I called the police, who, in turn, called the county ambulance, which took Jay to the hospital emergency room. Joe and I followed and then waited and waited and waited. Finally a doctor emerged. We followed him back to the treatment area, where I could see Jay lying motionless, eyes closed, with an intravenous tube in his arm. The doctor reported that Jay had a serious and life-threatening case of "aspirative pneumonia." In other words, food had gone down his windpipe and had entered his lungs instead of his stomach.

My memories tumbled over each other at top speed, at last making sense of this event. No wonder he had choked on his food. I had not yet seen the full meaning of this pneumonia, but I had come to see one explanatory connection.

The gravity of the situation hit me hard when the doctor asked if I would sign a "Do Not Resuscitate Order." Such an order asked that "heroic measures" not be taken to revive a patient in the event that his heart should stop. The doctors were asking me to agree that, if this should happen, they would not try to start Jay's heart again!

I began to realize that at times like this such momentous decisions were solely in the hands of a spouse, if there is one, and, if not, any close relative "responsible" for the patient's arrival at the hospital. It didn't seem right to me that a wife should have to put her name to her husband's death certificate. The doctor felt my reluctance and said quietly, almost gently, "I see that you think as I do. It is a tough thing to sign but there comes a time when the patient has had enough." Then he warned me that this may not be Jay's last pneumonia, that it might happen again, and that I was to be prepared.

No, I didn't know that it might happen again, because I had not yet seen the picture whole. Throughout Jay's ordeal, I was reacting to one isolated situation after another. There was no time to consider the whole picture; each portion was more than enough to handle. I thought of this pneumonia as an isolated and "chance" event. But in the light of the doctor's comment, I decided to sign. Having done so, I sat down, too washed out to stand. "A spouse is asked to be an executioner," I thought bitterly. I knew of Jay's deep fear of dying, which he understood to be "oblivion." I recalled signing my own "right to die" papers and carefully depositing them with my doctor and lawyer. That had only been a few years earlier, and, at the time, I wanted to raise the possibility with Jay. But since he was already ill, I felt that it was too late to bring up the issue. All I really wanted for Jay was that he die without pain and fear, a request easily accomplished by our modern drugs and tranquilizers—or so I thought.

The doctors worked over Jay and soon he responded to the antibiotics, as he typically did. After two weeks he was ready to return home. Life again seemed ready to resume its normal pace. But at the end of October, Joe knocked at my bedroom door, this time at one A.M. Jay had been coughing profusely and his fever was 105. I hastily dressed and we went through an exact duplication of last month's ordeal. Again, I signed a "DNR Order." Again, Jay responded and his second pneumonia backed off.

Jay's doctor wanted a conference with me. "This is the second trip within thirty days," he said, "you now have three options." First, I could take him home just as he is but in two weeks he will be back with another pneumonia, only this time he will be much weaker. Second, the hospital could put him on intravenous saline solution and add vitamins. But this meant that Jay would starve to death, and starvation is a very painful way to die. Finally, the doctors could put in a feeding tube and keep Jay going without repeated pneumonias.

The shock at being presented with this set of options was disorient-ing. I just couldn't think, and possibly that's why I didn't ask for some time to find out what some of the consequences of "enteral feeding" were, nor yet did I ask why death by starvation had to be painful. I was simply aghast at these equally objectionable alternatives. Could these be the *only* possible choices? Further, I became dimly aware that I was being asked, on the spot, to make a new and special kind of decision. I was being asked to decide whether Jay should live or die! I now knew this type of option-selection as "the caregiver's ultimate dilemma." I was being asked whether I was willing to accept for Jay this proposed new condition of life, about which I knew nothing. And I was being asked to make this decision right then and there. But how did I know what *he* would want? And would he want a feeding-tube-way-of-life in addition to all of his other travails and incapacities? Would all of this add up to an unacceptable situation for him? I looked at Jay, so helpless in his bed, and tried to put myself in his place. Sympathy poured over me like rain in a summer storm. I didn't really debate the issue, because it seemed to me that I had no alternative but to agree to tube feeding.

In passing, my attention focused on how thin Jay had become. He almost looked like the pictures I had seen of starving and dehydrated Africans. But what I hadn't noticed at the time was that no doctor had informed me of the problems he would face once the tube was in place. Nor did I know that the choice couldn't be retracted. Once in place, a feeding tube could not be removed without a court order, which was hard, if not impossible, to acquire. Once again I made an impossible decision, and again I was asked to sign a paper permitting some special procedure. I should have asked more questions. I should have known there would be problems. I should have. . . .

There are two kinds of mechanisms for machine feeding: one con-traption is put into the nostrils and down the esophagus; food is then delivered by this means to the stomach. Jay's condition couldn't sustain such an intrusive method. The chosen way for him was a rubber dome that would be implanted directly in his stomach. The dome would house and stabilize a rubber tube that pierced his stomach wall. At the exit site of the tube a second rubber dome would be placed over the opening, and out from it would come enough tubing to be attached to a feeding machine via a connection or "adapter."

The next time I saw Jay he was hooked up to a machine that held a bag containing a milky-white fluid. The machine was in motion because it was very accurately dispensing a certain number of drops per minute and propelling these into Jay's abdomen. Everything was measured and the machine was programmed to give him twelve hundred calories in twenty-four hours. Joe and I were given a briefing on how to care for Jay in his new machine-dependent state. At four-hour intervals, day and night, we were to open a fresh can of what looked and smelled like condensed milk. But before putting it in the food bag we were to hydrate Jay and clean the tube at the same time. This could be done by stopping the machine, opening the connection between Jay and the machine, and pouring one-half cup of room-temperature water down the tube. Then we were to reattach Jay to the machine and start it going again. It wasn't hard, but it was both tricky (in handling the machine) and demanding (in requiring both day and night attention). Not for a moment did I contemplate what kind of a life this would be for all three of us. At the time I saw no other available possibility.

Jay was brought home by ambulance; the machine, plus cases of food, had already been delivered by "the suppliers." An efficient young woman was on hand there to set up and program the machine and to give Joe and me new lessons because (of course) this machine operated differently than the one in the hospital.

At this point the hospital had already fitted Jay with an "indwelling" catheter, since a patient strapped to a feeding tube could not risk endangering the fragile connection to the life-giving machine by diaper changing. So now Jay lay on his hospital bed with his food hanging in a bag above and his urine going into a bag hanging below on the side of the bed. With all these impediments, tending to his wounds had been made very difficult, while turning him regularly was a genuine hassle. Both Joe and I were on twenty-four-hour duty. I was still teaching, so Joe was left on his own for a large part of the day.

This new situation brought problems that I, for one, had never dreamed of. Jay's mouth, no longer in use, had to be especially and painstakingly cared for. But again we were hosts to the visiting nurses, who showed themselves to be "skilled" in a very real sense. They demonstrated how to tend to his mouth with the aid of special swabs; how to tend his hair and skin, which now began to dry out rapidly; and how to move him, with all of the paraphernalia, into the living room. It is fortunate that all of these changes in Jay came on gradually over many years because it was hard to make an easy comparison between my tall, handsome husband of years past and this pathetically crippled invalid of the present. He had been so self-reliant and so dignified, so self-possessed and proud. It has been tough to confront all that has happened to that imperious autonomy. Only in retrospect was I able to piece together the various events that brought Jay to this point. It is odd how, when events take place over broad stretches of time, the mind tends to see them as separate and discrete rather than parts of an interconnected whole forming one series. For the first time I was able to connect Jay's mouth paralysis, when his tooth surgery occurred, to the paralysis of his lips when he couldn't get a spoon into his mouth because he couldn't find his mouth. In turn, this led to paralysis of his throat and his inability to correctly direct his swallowing into his esophagus. It had all been of a piece but I had been totally blind to it!

Life with a patient on a feeding tube is demanding, but Joe and I rose to the occasion. Since I had to get up early to leave for school, I took the midnight feeding while Joe took the four A.M. and eight A.M. feedings. Joe slept a bit during the afternoon, carefully setting his alarm so as not to miss a feeding. I, as always, did the food shopping on the way home, and then made dinner for Joe and me. Joe was actually on a nonstop twenty-four-hour service call but he never complained.

Thanksgiving was a very special time for us because we only had four close relatives and this was the only time of the year when we could all meet. Furthermore, Jay's sister, brother-in-law, and niece lived in northern New Jersey and our daughter was in south central Pennsylvania. To accommodate the distances that they had to travel and my teaching schedule, which gave me little time to prepare the dinner, we had made a tradition of celebrating the occasion on the Friday after Thanksgiving.

This year I was reluctant to even *try* to "celebrate" anything. Jay lay in his room, eyes closed, attached to a feeding tube. How could we bring him to the table to watch us enjoy food? Yet it didn't seem right to leave him in his room during the feast, either. The dilemma caused me to call off the family visit. Then I realized that Joe, who was staying over for the holiday, deserved a Thanksgiving dinner, especially since I knew that he regretted not having it with his wife and children. Habit took over and I prepared a small turkey for Joe and me. Then I couldn't eat a bit of it: empathy for Jay was having its way with me. How could I enjoy a holiday dinner without Jay being able to share it? I found holidays especially difficult during this stage of Jay's illness, not only because of the typical inability to get nursing help to relieve Joe but because a spirit of celebration was entirely out of keeping with my present life.

One of my conversations with Joe at dinner turned on America's technological society and its effect on the practice of medicine. I admired our fast-growing medical capability but distrusted it at the same time for turning individuals into machines and dehumanizing them. It viewed ailments as a mechanic puzzles over missing bolts, leaky hoses, and broken camshafts.

Joe commented on how different were American ways of treating the sick and the dying from those of his own culture, where, lacking technology, emphasis was on loving care. A dying person was surrounded by his children and relatives who cheered him on, comforting and caressing him. How different from being in a sterile hospital room surrounded only by strangers and machinery.

I agreed with Joe that treatment in the islands was so much more humane and that was what I really wanted for Jay. I wanted him to die peacefully without pain or fear. Surely, our advanced society could do this easily enough, but we simply don't want to. To "let" someone die in peace without rushing for any and all remedies that *might* maintain minimal life is foreign to our way of thinking and that of our medical community. And it was to me as well. It seems that we have to *do* something and not just sit still and let things happen. I was reminded of a beautiful old Negro spiritual that encourages the surrounding company to *help* the victim die. "Walk him up the Stairs" (to the Pearly Gates), it commanded. "Push him up the hill," it urged, and then "Help him out the door."

Between Thanksgiving and Christmas Joe and I began to have troubles for which neither of us had been prepared. Although we followed the assigned routine without fail, Jay's feeding tube kept getting stopped up. After many efforts to clear it, I called his doctor. "Bring him to the hospital," he said. The ambulances in my area charge $350 for a two-mile round trip. I felt that the matter should have been resolved more easily and less expensively. Medicare doesn't pay for ambulances and after further thought about the hassle it would be to transport Jay each time his feeding tube clogged, I turned to our friends, the local police, who, by this time, were quite aware of our situation. They had an idea. On the county ambulances there were at least two paramedics who were experienced in solving this particular problem. The police would send us help! Shortly thereafter, when a county ambulance stopped in front of our house, we were jubilant. A paramedic bent over Jay and got straight to work. I didn't see what he was doing but Joe, two other ambulance attendants, and I waited breathlessly around the bed. When the paramedic stood up and announced, "It's clear," a cheer went up from the observers. What kind of thanks does one give such unknown and unrecognized heroes for their dedication?

Not long after the feeding tube incident, Joe told me that the adapter (the connection between Jay and the feeding machine) was cracked and leaking badly. It was soaking the bed. I rushed to the hospital and brought home an adapter. It didn't fit! Exasperated, we stopped the machine and I cut off the offending connection in order to take it with me as an aid in finding its mate. It was a daring move since, were I not to find a solution, Jay would have to return to the hospital to have an operation to reseat the tube. The hospital that had installed the tube in the first place had no such connector. The doctor hadn't recorded the number or the manufacturer on Jay's chart. Desperate, I rushed to two other hospitals in the area but *no one* could find an appropriate fitting!

First, panic set in. But then my anger and anxiety blended into a real witch's brew. How could this be? I frantically drove back to the hospital where the job had been done and shouted that I would not leave until they supplied me with some sort of workable connection. A nurse came hastily, examined the offending piece of technology and commented: "The tubing put in is *not* feeding tubing but catheter tubing!" In a low voice she told me that "operating doctors sometimes just grab anything in sight." She darted away and returned with new connection materials: on one side was feeding tubing, on the other catheter tubing. Makeshift, to say the least, but it worked.

When I used to fantasize about keeping Jay at home until he died, I had a peaceful image of a bedridden patient who would require much less care than a wobbly ambulatory one. The exact opposite was the case. Little did I know that a bed-bound patient had to be turned every two hours at the very least and preferably once an hour. "Turning" is easier said than done, believe me. But there are techniques. A "draw-sheet" (a sheet folded crossways into a two- or three-foot-wide piece) is placed across the bed approximately where the patient's buttocks would be. Then two attendants, standing on either side of the bed, would grasp either side of the rig. One would use this leverage to push while the other pulled. With considerable effort on the part of *both* attendants, the patient could be rolled from one side to the other. This maneuver obviously involved a nursing crew. Changing sheets while the patient was in bed proved to be such an arduous task that we found it worth the extra effort to avoid it as much as possible. Instead, Jay could be lifted, tubing and all, into a wheelchair during the short time it took to change sheets; then he was lifted back into bed.

Christmas and New Year's found me once more struggling to find help in order to provide some relief for Joe. As usual there was not a chance, because New York State, in all of its legislative wisdom, passed a law that, at minimum, "Licensed Practical Nurses" had the legal right to tend a patient on a feeding tube! I called several agencies, but they had no nurses available until after the holidays. Of course, with this encouragement from the state, their salary had not only increased to $30 per hour (from $10) but now they would not work a twenty-four-hour day but only for ten hours each day! Not only would I need two such nurses—one for the day and one for the night—but I would still be left with a four-hour period every twenty-four hours when I would have no nursing help at all! Joe volunteered to stay on during the holidays, but he was as exhausted as I was.

At this point I was finally ready to throw in the towel. While I wasn't one to give up easily on anything, the obstacles had become so numerous and so overwhelming that this seemed to be a good time to give up. I reluctantly and angrily admitted that I couldn't deal with multiple problems, none of which had a solution.

Having admitted this, what was I to do? I knew that no nursing home was willing to take Jay even *before* he needed this present level of care. This avenue was closed, except, perhaps, had he been a Medicaid patient for whom there are always public resources and homes to be tapped. The "private" patient (who can pay) can be turned down by nursing homes, and we had no access to public facilities!

Looking back on it I realize that once a loved one is no longer ambulatory (in other words, permanently bedridden), home care is indeed very difficult. But if life-sustaining machinery is also in place, home care is suicidal madness. Machinery tends to be cussed at best and requires constant attention day and night. Only a staff of many who can spell one another is able to monitor adequately a feeding machine serving a totally inert patient. However, it is well not to wait too long. It is better to move to institutional care when machine therapy is only a likely prospect since this level of care frightens many nursing homes. And so again I found myself without a single viable option that would permit any throwing in of towels. The red, sandpapered blotches made a return visit.

7

A Nursing Home: Down for the Count (1989)

I faced the New Year 1989 dazed, angry, frustrated, and confused. At least the next couple of weeks would be less hectic. The University's intersession relieved me of having to think about committee meetings, budgets, teaching, and grading examinations and papers. My head was so filled with Jay that I had room for little else. Having reached one dead end after another in my search for some viable solution to the "problem with Jay," I *couldn't* think—not one more thought. Jay could no longer stay at home, yet nursing homes wouldn't take him with his bedsores, hospitals had no place for those with no chance of being healed and discharged, and there were no hospices for this type of protracted dying.

Immediately after New Year's Day, the visiting nurses again made a welcome appearance. I needed both counsel and comfort and they were especially good at both. This time, however, they had bad news. The extent of Jay's sores had reached serious if not life-threatening proportions. The tissue had so degenerated that hospital attention was needed. Furthermore, his arms and one shoulder now showed signs of tissue breakdown —the organisms were migrating. The nurses sent their carefully prepared report to Jay's doctor, who suggested that I make an appointment at the hospital's newly instituted "Wound Center," which was devoted to tending to all varieties of sores that refused to heal, regardless of treatment or care.

On a cold day in the middle of January we bundled Jay up and Joe carried him to the car. As we wheeled Jay from the elevator to one of the hospital offices, I happened to turn to look at him. Jay's straggly, uncut hair dangled from beneath the back of his fur hat, his mouth was hanging open crookedly; his eyes seemed to stare straight ahead, empty and unfocused; and his jacket was misbuttoned. Jay looked demented, unkempt, and in clothes three sizes too large for him. He could easily have been mistaken for a derelict from a homeless shelter. What a sorry spectacle. How he would have shuddered at the sight of himself! I tried to make light of it, commenting that a bedridden patient could hardly look chic, but I was too pained with empathy for him to carry it off.

Emerging from the examining room, Joe wrestled Jay into his jacket. The doctor wanted to speak to me. I could feel the necessity of another decision coming on and I felt that all-too-familiar pressure that consumed me when I had to decide virtually on the spot what to do for Jay.

The doctor was a "wound specialist" who had moved from England to head the new center. He supplied me with articles he had written on the subject (complete with pictures and diagrams of various types of ancillary surgery), all of which seemed to me to be quite innovative. At least he had ideas. He wanted Jay to be immediately admitted to the hospital, and I readily concurred. My dilemma concerning how best to care for Jay was to be settled, at least for the time being. As that unbelievable fact began to sink in, I felt almost elated. I filled out the many papers required to gain admittance to the facility. How many times had I filled out forms of one kind or another. It seemed I had left a paper trail that would stretch for miles. And now, miracle of miracles, here was Doctor X, who actually proposed a treatment regimen for Jay's devil sores. No more medical hand wringing; I was going to see some action.

That first night, as I sat alone, I experienced the fullest extent of my relief from Jay's insoluable problems. I was deeply grateful that he was not only in good hands but that something was finally going to be done to battle those damned sores. At least *something* was going to be done!

The change of residence from home to hospital as well as the change of doctors made Jay much more alert than he had been at home. I was soon to realize the reason. The doctor was coming several times a week to "debride" him; that is, the doctor was in the process of cutting out the dead tissue from Jay's wounds. I noticed signs in the room urging hand-washing if one touched the patient anywhere, pointing out that this was not because of what the visitor could do to the patient but what the patient could do to the visitor! I was informed by the nurses and staff that Jay's wounds were highly toxic. I noticed that nurses threw away many pairs of rubber gloves in the process of dressing his wounds, and there was a warning in the hall about the entire area being toxic. And I saw that when they treated the now deepened wounds with some type of power spray, they carried off the liquid in covered basins.

Jay had been assigned a special bed in a room equipped with special electrical outlets. I had been told that the bed would remove the pressure on all parts of his body and that he would feel as if he were floating on air. The bed was a formidable sight indeed. When I came into the room I couldn't see Jay at all. Instead, I saw a supersized oval steel tub sitting on a high platform that appeared to house its internal parts, or so I gathered from the look of the colored lights, dials, and knobs. It reminded me of a large, padded casket. In order to get a glimpse of Jay, I had to mount a platform that surrounded the entire contraption. Though I didn't realize it at the time, probably because I was busy reading the literature that hung beside the bed, this therapeutic bed was to put an end to my sitting close to Jay and holding his hand, activities that I found reassuring and I suspect that he did, too, were he aware enough to notice them.

Jay was positioned deep within this monster, resting on what looked like rubber sheeting that was bouncing around. Tiny pellets were being bombarded from underneath the rubber and these pellets relieved pressure on his entire body. I was told that at no time would his own weight exert pressure on his bedsores, except for a moment or two. The air in the room was in motion, too, as if a huge fan were blowing. It made a whirring sound, and I could feel the room air drying out my own skin.

The doctor explained what he intended to do. He was going to remove all of Jay's infected tissue, then replace it first with grafts of adjacent muscle, to be followed by grafts of skin from his thighs. I remembered seeing a picture of this in one of the brochures that the doctor had given me and was horrified at the prospect. When completed, the reconstructed area was hideous looking, revoltingly bumpy and uneven. I wondered whether anyone would be able to sit again after such a process. The more I thought about the surgery, the more sure I became that I would reject this route. The doctor would have to find another patient on whom to display the procedure to a bevy of admiring interns.

The bedsore on Jay's right hip had not only penetrated to the bone, but spread to the area underneath. The bone obscured the staff's view of the sore, obliging the surgeon to use merely his hands to blindly determine good from bad tissue. I decided to see the wound for myself. The doctor looked surprised: "Are you *sure*?" My resounding affirmation brought action. Jay's tissue had been removed, leaving a wide and deep hole. I saw the whitish bone and a pink-grey muscle through the bright red meat of the surrounding tissue. I gathered that this was the muscle the doctor had planned to provide with a new job.

I couldn't help but wonder whether we should be subjecting Jay to all of this. Was it really necessary? How did it feel? He didn't seem to be in pain. I kept telling myself that what was removed had been diseased tissue that could have eventually poisoned his entire body. That thought made me acknowledge the *only* move I was totally unwilling to make. I just couldn't put Jay through the ordeal of a muscle transplant.

The day after I had refused the surgery, the hospital, much to my horror, downgraded Jay's "skilled care" condition to "intermediate care," which, in his case, was woefully inadequate. This was cruel, I thought. I wanted an explanation. The hospital was obviously going to discharge him. The "discharge planner" to whom I had been sent said something about a "misunderstanding" between the surgeon and me. I told her that I hadn't known of any such thing and wanted to know what this was all about. I wondered how much pressure they would put on me to extract a positive decision. While I was repulsed by the proposed procedure, what would we do with an open hole?

The medical tribe, it seems, can be masters of evasion. I certainly was getting a double helping. When I asked about Jay's prognosis, the doctor replied, "I'm not God." Would nursing homes be more or less likely to take him in this condition? The doctor was rather dismissive: "That's not my department, ask the discharge planner." I did, and her answer was, "I can't make a decision for you." Desperately seeking to escape this irrelevance, I turned again to the doctor: "Will recuperation from this surgery (the muscle transplant) be painful?" The answer: "They seldom feel much pain in this state." Then I asked, "Will he be able to sit up comfortably?" Answer: "Some do and some don't."

At this point, I was so concerned about the "intermediate" care to which this deeply ill man was being subjected that I was about to boil over with exasperation. I asked the discharge planner what would happen were I to flatly refuse the muscle operation (I was still on the fence about it even though my back was to the wall). She countered with the first straight and nonevasive answer: "We would look for the first nursing home that would take him." Then I asked whether he would get the same intermediate care from the hospital until such time as they found a nursing home. "There is nothing further we can do for him," I was told. Would the hospital summarily discharge Jay? No, but he would no longer be using (though it was more likely that they would not be extending) the full facilities of the hospital.

Meantime, after repeated attempts to contact the surgeon, I was finally granted an audience. In one of the brochures he had given me, I read about an interesting new treatment, so I came directly to the point. I wanted to try Procuran to promote healing and the growth of new tissue. I don't know just where or how the idea of Procuran originated, but it seems that our surgeon either developed it or had a hand in the research. I didn't dare ask lest such a question would interfere with the cooperative atmosphere I was now enjoying.

Procuran is a curative substance developed from a patient's own blood cells. The procedure calls for blood to be drawn and sent to a laboratory where the "fighter" and "healer" cells are separated out. These cells are then cultured and artificially grown until a sufficient volume of them have been produced. A lotion made of these cells is applied to the patient's wounds. In other words, this innovative procedure would use the patient's own blood to come to his aid. The idea fascinated me with its possibilities of treating many sorts of ailments.

The doctor was warm and hospitable but warned me that therapy with Procuran was costly: around a thousand dollars per month for its production and use. I told him that I would leave a check for it at the desk on the way out. Then he further reminded me that Medicare would not pay for the therapy: "Medicare has not yet been educated to this idea, but we are trying." Medicare had been paying for Jay's hospital stay all along, so I felt that I could afford this radical new treatment. I also demanded that Jay be immediately returned to skilled nursing care status. He was.

The treatment produced by the Procuran therapy was nothing short of an absolute miracle. Once a week I would be shown the wounds and each time a quarter inch or so of new healthy tissue was growing back where infection and decay had once taken root. Jay's own personal medicine was healing both the sores and his deep wound. I could not believe my eyes. Elated and excited, I spoke to the surgeon about the possibility of using this method for healing other types of ailments: for example, burns or leprosy, where flesh becomes putrefied. He agreed that Procuran was showing considerable promise.

When Jay's own healthy tissue reached the level of his outer skin, grafts were taken from his thighs and put on the raw opening. Jay had been in the hospital for almost five months and the staff felt that they had done just about all they could. It was time to leave. But now, with his bedsores a thing of the past, I was no longer in doubt about finding Jay a nursing home.

I started my search for a home, aided by the hospital discharge planner. Homes are categorized according to the different levels of care they provide. The facilities that are typically called "Retirement Villages" or "communities" are not really nursing homes; rather, they are clusters of small independent living units or one large apartment building for congregate living. All provide an optional meal service and some have nursing facilities affiliated with them for those who become temporarily ill. Most of these homes are inhabited by reasonably well-to-do persons in their sixties or early seventies who want to be independent of their children but do not want to live alone. They are hotels for the ambulatory elderly who prefer the companionship of older adults to babysitting for their grandchildren. Many residents keep and use their own cars. While all homes typically provide scheduled events, entertainments, amusements, shops and beauty salons, these homes are designed to meet the needs of the active and relatively healthy.

Some older adults are in need of help with bathing, dressing, medication, and the basic tasks of living. Here the facility's care is primarily custodial, with events and activities appropriate to the residents' capabilities. Every nursing home is concerned with what they call the "quality of life" of their clients. Some really work at this aspect of elder care, compiling reports and conducting meetings about what the facility is providing and should provide for each inhabitant. All nursing homes display bulletin boards announcing the daily fare of amusements and activities.

As the elderly become more debilitated, a "skilled nursing facility" may be needed. With twenty-four-hour nursing staff, these homes are capable of providing many of the treatments and techniques that hospitals offer. Most nursing homes are eager to maintain a balance between residents who are in need of immediate care and those in the skilled nursing unit who require infinitely more care at an increasingly higher cost. There are facilities that serve all levels of care, which seems to be a trend for the future of this growing segment of the health-care industry. Furthermore, some homes have "physical therapy and rehabilitation" units attached to them. In the case of stroke patients these services can be a tremendous help.

There is nothing more intensive than skilled care for the totally incapacitated, those who suffer from chronic illness, or the dying. At present, there is no suitable type of facility geared to the needs of Parkinson's patients, Alzheimer's victims, those who have suffered multiple strokes, or anyone in the last stages of a debilitating disease. Hospice treatment for the terminally ill remains focused on cancer patients, though some facilities have begun to open their doors to AIDS patients. Hospice care consists primarily in relief of pain, psychological aid, and strong doses of tenderness. As the numbers of those with chronic debilitating disease increase, the need to develop hospice-like care for patients whose dying is protracted would go far toward lightening both the financial and psychological burdens that mates and relatives must shoulder.

The earlier apprehension voiced by many skilled care facilities I had contacted concerning admitting Jay had appeared to evaporate, for within a day of beginning our search, the discharge planner (who is, incidentally, a relatively new and welcome member of the hospital staff) found a nearby nursing home and recommended it highly as being one of the finest. It should be, I gasped, upon hearing that the *base* price for a bed and care was well over five thousand dollars a month! *Basic care* does not include doctor visits by house physicians retained by the facility to make both regular monthly visits and answer emergency calls. It also does not include medications (prescription or nonprescription), laundry service, hair care, or the host of paraphernalia needed to help prevent skin abrasion and its frequent accompaniment, bedsores. Residents were expected to pay extra for bandages, antiseptics, lotions, salves, nurses gloves, and other materials used in the sick room. Most nursing homes do provide some level of physical therapy, which is typically recommended for stroke patients, but it, too, is not included in the room fee. Furthermore, in our case, there was the added expense of renting a feeding machine and buying the canned food. In short, the total bill for care during just one month's stay could easily double the original room and care fee! Jay needed this intensive care but how were we going to pay for it?

As fate would have it, the U.S. Congress had just passed its "Catastrophic Health Care Act," which entitled Jay to five full months of care at approximately half the cost I had been quoted. The premiums older Americans had to pay for this coverage were substantial. This, however, did not alter the home's policy of requiring a fifteen-thousand-dollar deposit before Jay could enter its doors! This amount was to be held in escrow to be used if and when we had to move to another home because we could no longer pay the monthly fees. I doubt that those who subsequently eliminated the Catastrophic Health Care Act on the grounds that its premiums were too high had even the faintest notion regarding the price of nursing home care in metropolitan areas.

I knew that this solution was only stop-gap, a way of biding our time while I looked in other states for a suitable nursing home. Up to the point at which the feeding tube was installed, I could take care of Jay at home, and his own income was adequate to see to his needs. I had to keep a very close watch on expenditures since I, too, was now retired and had to consider my needs and the upkeep of our homes. I thought long and hard about selling the Vermont farm, but that just didn't seem right since our daughter had asked only for that as her inheritance. I considered taking a mortgage on our house in New York, but it didn't take much calculation to realize that Jay's nursing home bills alone would consume the equity in our home in no time. Nor did it seem right that everything Jay and I had worked for was about to go up in smoke. If Jay had any real chance for a life, I would surely have pursued one of these options. As it turned out, there simply was no painless solution in sight.

I became exhausted, depressed, and then angry at our fate. At times my anger was directed at Jay. Why did he persist in "living," if you could call his semi-comatose state life? The question brought on a real evaluation of his "quality of life" rather than retreating to my usual (and unexamined) view that *human* life had to be preserved, even if it was comatose. His quality of life was nil: he showed no sign of recognition of me or anyone around him, and his eyes were typically closed. I wished that he would die! Why didn't he just go? Guilt surrounded by empathy set in and I hated myself for what I was thinking. What if our positions had been reversed? In spite of my personal commitment to the "right to die," how would I feel if he wished a similar fate for me had I been under his care?

I tried to clarify my thoughts but to no avail. We were moving Jay into the nursing home and I was in his room awaiting the ambulance attendants who were bringing him. They arrived in great haste, picked him up off the gurney in a sheet and threw him on the bed. I felt apprehension immediately and, sure enough, when we pulled out the sheet from under him, it was covered with hard, steel sutures! I hadn't known that this suturing was so recent. Apparently, none of the nurses at the hospital had either the good will or presence of mind to ask that he be put down gently.

I knew what this meant; I knew that all of those months in the hospital were about to be undone. Early on, Jay's long-time doctor had commented on the debriding: "The trouble with the procedure is that the grafts don't take and it all starts over again." In my mind's eye I saw the deep hole and the ivory bone again.

It was then that I made a new discovery. Jay lay in a fetal position. I asked the nursing home staff to stretch him out so that he would lie more comfortably. The nurse turned to me and said, "His muscles are permanently constricted." I tried to grasp the meaning of this since I had never heard of such a thing before.

"What do you mean by 'permanently'?" I asked.

"He will never be able to move his muscles from that position again!"

In other words, Jay was frozen in place for a lifetime—or whatever was left of it. Of all of his troubles, this one hit me particularly hard. I had never heard of muscle constriction. I tried to overcome my disbelief.

I immediately saw the new changes now to come in his life. He could never again sit up, anywhere—in bed, in a wheelchair, or in a "gerichair" designed for stretched-out legs. He was not just an invalid unable to walk; he was totally incapable of bodily movement either by his own initiative or through the manipulation of others. He had to remain lying down for the rest of his life.

"Oh my God," was all I could say before I turned from the scene and rushed to the car, which I always did when overcome by horror and grief. I couldn't absorb what I saw or let myself acknowledge what I knew. If there ever was a contemporary Gethsemane, it is the plight of a burned-out caregiver, too exhausted and beset with troubles to face one more problem; one who is too empathic to see her charge lose every single capacity, one by one, until nothing is left.

My thoughts returned to the hospital. They had made no attempt to bring physical therapists to the scene. No mention was made of this possibility, which I might have been able to prevent or at least forestall had I only known. There was more evidence that a hospital was not the place for Jay. On one occasion I noticed that Jay's plastic food bag was filled with water rather than food. I surmised that the "wound" nurses were impatient with the repeated care of the feeding tube and decided to save time by hydrating him all at once. I said nothing because I couldn't believe my reasoning was correct. A day or two later, at six in the morning, an intern whose English had an oriental sound, informed me that Jay's feeding tube had clogged and that the intern had tried to free it with a wire but that he had accidentally lost hold of the wire, dropping it into Jay's abdomen! He continued by reassuring me that while he had succeeded in retrieving the wire, he had, in the process, dislodged the internal dome in Jay's stomach! They weren't able to retrieve the dome so they seated a new one! I sensed that I had been told all this to prevent a malpractice suit, since they were admitting that an accident had occurred.

I rushed to the hospital and asked whether there was reason to believe that the wire might have torn his stomach lining and caused internal bleeding. The hospital responded matter-of-factly that they had already taken care of that possibility by giving him a blood transfusion! I asked what they proposed to do about the lost dome. Their response was that it couldn't be seen by X-ray and that it would either be passed through the colon or Jay's stomach acids would eventually dissolve it!

I realized that I had already known of this type of hospital behavior when I sent my private duty nurse Joe to wash and cut Jay's hair, to trim his nails, and to give him a shave, since Jay had become more and more unkempt. Perhaps this is not so strange. Jay was in the hospital for wounds, and wounds were all they saw or tended to in the ward to which he was assigned. The results of overspecialization were obvious. The staff totally overlooked *the patient* and his *other needs* in the process! After all, a hospital is given to specialization and short-term stays. Typically, a hospitalized patient can either take care of his own needs or declare them to his nurses. It is easy for a caregiver to overlook the fact that there is some hazard in taking an elderly stroke victim to the hospital for a specialized, albeit related, illness since a hospital is not a nursing home. Only a nursing home is oriented to "seeing the patient whole"—seeing his or her many illnesses and incapacities individually as well as being interrelated. Only a nursing home is alert to the many things that can happen to an elderly person. Only a nursing home has the time to take stock of both physical and emotional needs. Sometimes a nursing home is the only plausible place left to obtain care for the stroke patient, regardless of how guilty caregivers feel about authorizing the placement or how much they blame their own deficiencies and inabilities.

The money problem continued to haunt me. My sister in Georgia scouted the area and sent brochures of nursing homes there. I traveled to Vermont and searched. Our daughter duplicated the quest in her small town in Pennsylvania. In all three states, what seemed to be skilled and efficient homes were less than half what residents in New York were expected to pay, sometimes much less.

Of all the voices, our daughter's was the strongest and most insistent. Between her work in television, radio, and newspapers, she rarely had a chance to come home during her father's long illness. The media knows no holidays and respects them even less. She pleaded with me to place Jay in a home near her on the grounds that she never had a proper chance to tell him how much she appreciated him. She wanted to stand in for me, to give me a rest, and do her part.

I traveled to the charming old town that housed the college from which she and I had graduated. I found myself sitting by the little river on the campus where, forty-nine years earlier, I had agreed to marry Jay, over my parents' objections. Memories crowded in. The town boasted a Mennonite nursing home, which peaked my curiosity. After all, my ancestors were Mennonites who had come to this country from Switzerland and settled in the area some fifty years before the Revolution in order to escape religious persecution.

The Mennonite home was spread over many acres of land and built on three layers of hills. There was an "independent living" area on the lowest level, with little four-room bungalows complete with backyard porches, picnic grills, flower gardens and grassy lawns, and a parking bay in front. An in-coming resident would buy one of these homes by putting down approximately what one year of nursing home care would cost on Long Island. This paid completely for the home, making it rent free from there on. When independent living was no longer possible and institutional care was needed, the home was resold to a new resident (there is a long waiting list) with the proceeds going toward the nursing care of the previous owner. It looked to me like one of the best solutions to senior care I have ever seen.

The second layer of hills provided "intermediate" nursing care. Here patients were provided with whatever aid they needed in living. At the top level was a large double-winged structure that dominated the whole scene. This was the "skilled nursing" area. It was spacious, quiet, peaceful, immaculately maintained, and beautiful. I was given a tour and taken to the area for the very ill. This was in one of the two wings. The second wing, far removed from the first, housed the pounding and swearing Alzheimer's patients. The home did not put these two types of patients together, as is often done in New York. Here tender loving care could be provided much like in a hospice. I looked in several rooms. In the first I saw white mesh-capped Mennonite women tending a patient. The next room revealed another Mennonite nurse sitting quietly, holding her patient's hand. For the Mennonites, nursing is a "mission," a "calling," a kind of ministry. I knew that they understood nursing to be a direct command from God to give their lives to the gentle care of the sick. I went out to the rose garden (roses, roses everywhere) and sat down on the earth beside them. I had come home and I knew it. Between this mountain ridge and that, I would bring my dying husband to what was ultimately my own homeland and where I believed in the integrity of the people.

But this was not to be. The Mennonite home had special obligations, not only to those who inhabited other parts of the complex but also to the community at large. Someone had suddenly become ill and needed the bed that had been reserved for Jay. The home suggested that I go to "the other" home in the community, which they recommended, but warmly and hospitably suggested that we could return when there was room if we wished.

The "other" home in this historic town was founded by and named for a former governor of the state. It, too, turned out to be unlike anything I had ever seen before. It was both attractive *and* technologically sophisticated, boasting the only "rehabilitation" center for miles around. Immaculate, as usual, its single-story building spread out in a starlike pattern. The spaces outside between the segments of the star had secluded areas where patients and guests could sit. All rooms had views either of neatly kept private homes or a thriving cornfield. Capped secular nurses mingled with the mesh-capped Mennonite ones. Its small, intimate, and homelike dining rooms boasted colorful tablecloths with thick plastic covers to fit. Little bouquets of flowers decorated each table. Some diners were gingerly manipulating forks; others sat placidly while white-clad aides fed them. Here and there interspersed throughout the facility were little parlors where small groups watched television or played cards. There was a small and lovely chapel and, at each apex of the star, there were "guest parlors" where patients could bring guests to sit and relax. The one near Jay's room had a fireplace with a gas-burning flame leaping over artificial logs. These were cozy and warm spots that bolstered the spirit. Everything was carpeted and curtained.

There was surely nothing "institutional" about this place, even though the several "nurse's stations" were efficiently busy with keeping records and answering patients' bells. The atmosphere of the home was so entirely different from any I had encountered in New York that I asked if they had a room for Jay. They did. It might be worth noting that neither of these homes asked for a complete history of Jay's condition in order to decide whether or not they would take him. Since I didn't want them to be shocked when they examined Jay, I volunteered just how seriously ill he was. The response was so warm and friendly: "It sounds as if he needs us and we are both happy and well-prepared to take care of him."

I took the room at once. It was a very large, bright room with three other bedded-down men. The home felt that Jay needed company, and he would always be watched since there was a nurse there regularly, caring for one man or another. The basic cost of this very pleasant place was *exactly half* of the expected cost for similar accommodations and care in New York! Our daughter lived but five minutes away and her best friend, who had also volunteered to oversee matters, had been a nurse's aide at the home. My trip back to New York was devoted to trying to digest just what I had done.

I told our mutual friends about the move. To my astonishment they were critical and almost hostile. "You are too concerned with money." "You're stingy with him. Why didn't you mortgage the house?" "You're taking him away from us so we can no longer see him." And, worse, still, "You are pushing him away, trying to get rid of him." I concluded that there was no way I could make them to understand the many and varied considerations that went into my decision. Perhaps no one can understand the web of meanings, memories, and interconnections that make up an individual life; and perhaps no one should be expected to. I granted them the right to come to their own conclusions because, for the first time, I stood my ground.

The long-distance ambulance collected the seventeen hundred dollars in cash. New York, I guess, will always be true to form. Maybe it is just what urban life is and perhaps has to be. The driver and the paramedic loaded Jay aboard and I watched the ambulance move slowly out of the hospital parking lot. It's brake light went on as it waited at the exit for a car to pass. As it disappeared around the corner for its very long journey with Jay, helpless and totally at my mercy, I started the car. But my head, unable to be commanded, went down on the steering wheel in exhaustion, depletion, and sorrow.

As I turned into the driveway of the home that Jay and I had built together, I realized that he would never again enter its door. The impact of what I had done was only beginning to sink in. Up to this point I had so much on my mind that it diverted my attention from the meaning of what I was doing. I was alone, a widow for all intents and purposes, yet so deeply involved with Jay. (Was he all right in the ambulance?)

Our daughter was on the phone. She was waiting for the ambulance when it arrived. As they brought the stretcher out, his eyes were open and the attendants stopped to let father and daughter greet one another. As they stared at each other, a slight smile of recognition passed over Jay's face. She kissed him and he returned to sleep, feeling safe again. I hung up and listened to the silence of the house.

8

A Report on the Condition of the Arena

JAY IN PENNSYLVANIA

The out-of-state nursing home turned out to be as I had expected—dedicated, knowledgeable, and efficient. The staff accepted Jay graciously without complaining about his especially deteriorated condition. They promptly took photos of Jay's bedsores in order to measure their own progress in healing them with their own methods. Lack of care in the New York home had indeed returned his sores to their original condition. His tissue was again destroyed to the bone and the new home had to start again from scratch, but this time without the hospital, its debriding surgeon, and the miracle healing agent Procuran. No laboratory in the area was equipped to convert his blood into the healing lotion. Jay had to go along with whatever local ingenuity could provide. However, I was comforted to know that his nerve endings at the site of the sores had long ago been destroyed and that he felt no pain whether the sores healed or not.

The home did request, however, that we again put him on the special air-cushion bed, which, of course, would return his expenses to almost double his income, and this I had wanted to avoid. Seeing my indecision about the bed, the home brought on a typical American deal: if I would buy the bed for two months (a mere six thousand dollars), the company would give me the third month free! I took them up on the deal as a recognition of their resolve to push the devil sores back to a manageable distance.

Their methods consisted in an almost continuous flow of care with salves, creams, and antiseptic washes, augmented by frequent turning of his body, manually exercising his arms and legs, and using electronic massage on his hips. It worked! In time the smaller sore healed entirely while the large one, which had been surgically treated, ended up needing only a final layer of tissue to totally heal. I recalled that Jay's physician had told me that the final layer was the most difficult and problematic; it usually never healed since grafts often didn't "take." However, the new nurses had been right. Bedsores do indeed result from a lack of care.

This attention to his body, however, had no effect on his mind, which seemed to move further and further away from events around him. It moved "in" and "out" unpredictably and often in quick alteration. Sometimes he would look at me when I spoke to him but at other times he would look at the corner of the room, apparently neither seeing nor hearing me. I found it increasingly difficult to avoid feeling disappointed and frustrated—even snubbed and spurned. I had made such a long and arduous journey to let him know that I cared and it was hard to be reconciled to this unpredictable mindlessness without feeling profound futility and, yes, anger. At such times I would typically take refuge in the car. In the space that I had carved out for "me" I would try to gain some kind of perspective on the emotional storm whirling around me. I was beginning to accept the fact that Jay was now beyond help and that I was about to enter a new plateau of life—widowhood. I used to have a clear sense of Jay's "presence"—that he was in some sense "there," even when we were so far apart—but now, his essence, what made him who he was, had begun to recede and I wasn't yet fully reconciled to it.

No wonder I didn't want to sell the car! It had been through so much of this illness with us. It took us to his many doctors; it was in this very car that Jay spilled the coffee, as if to underline the information of the neurologist that the CAT scan had revealed his brain to be increasingly scarred. This insistent return to the past put in sharp relief the difference between what he once was and what he had now become. I remembered that when I bought the car I took him to the dealer's lot to see it. He approved with enthusiasm and named it "Lummette" as a proper mate to his big wagon, which he had dubbed "Lummox." When I drove into our Vermont driveway last year a neighbor commented quizzically, "I see that you are still driving your old wagon." To which I replied, "You had better get used to it since I have a special connection with it." Strange how things can get so entwined with one's life that they encapsulate a whole range of memories.

The trip down memory lane brought me to another scene that I now regard with some irony. In the early days of our marriage, when we had spoken of such things as insurance and wills, I apparently had a fixed image of death, which was that I (and most everyone) would drop dead in my (their) tracks. The Grim Reaper simply crept up from behind and with one blow put an end to life—D.O.A. I had no conception of the type of dying that was indefinitely protracted over many years. Nor did I know about a gradual but steady loss of capacities that we identify with "living." I surely didn't imagine the possibility that each loss of capacity brought troublesome empathy and pain to a spouse. Of all the ways for a mate to die, the protracted one is the most arduous. Crises are always turning up, new losses are always quietly mourned, and new forebodings for the future are always threatening. When a mate dies suddenly, the survivor is intensely shocked to begin with, but each subsequent day can bring some alleviation through new adjustments. In protracted dying, however, while there are shocks as the illness irrevocably progresses, these fade into an ever-increasing exhaustion and weariness, heavily overlaid with anger and sorrow. One gradually realizes that there is no reprieve for the inevitable event yet to come. It ominously lurks in the wings, to be confronted.

However, Jay's life in the new nursing home was far from dull. Although I was too often absent, students and friends seemed willing to make the long trip to see him. My "honorary daughter," Gail, visited several times a week, often bringing her eight-year-old daughter, Jasmine, with her. Meantime, life had indeed moved on. Our daughter had decided to marry and our future son-in-law, eight years her senior, brought with him, from a previous marriage, three beautiful children, ages six, eleven, and sixteen respectively. "My tribe" had indeed increased. Four children now called us "Grandma" and "Grandpa." I believe that it was this cluster of children that most interested Jay. The four visited him separately and as a group, being allowed to softly sing, dance, and recite for him. The scene was lively, a far cry from the sterile and monotonous atmosphere of the New York nursing home. Jay's bedside bulletin board was laden with many versions of "I love you, Grandpa," each decorated with its own drawings. On his special pressure-relieving bed, Jay could most effortlessly see the ceiling, which was kept decorated with clusters of colored helium balloons, and some mobiles that fluttered with the slightest breeze. While no one knew how much of this Jay understood, it didn't really matter. He seemed most alert when the children were with him, keeping his eyes open and following the action. Here and there it was reported that he smiled. The children seemed to take Jay's illness for granted, being innocent of its ominous implications.

Now, at this point in time, Jay's sores had been so very much relieved that we (the nursing home staff and I) decided to substitute a regular bed for the pressure-relieving one, thus, for the first time, putting Jay's expenses back within his income. Within a week, both bedsores had reopened. And again they requested a return to the expensive bed. It looked as if I would never be relieved of this excessive financial burden. This was now a well-traveled road, and I felt my resistance rising. His care had been so incredibly expensive that I had already gone deep into our savings. It seemed unfair that having made this move to another state to avoid impoverishing expenses, the high cost of care nonetheless turned up again and again in this new setting.

Furthermore, for the first time I began receiving bills for 20 percent of the rental for the feeding machine and the food. No one had asked for this previously and, since his life depended on it, Medicare had always taken care of the cost. And it seemed that *again* I was to have dealings with "the suppliers" with whom I had experience when Jay was at home. This particular medical support group seems to enjoy an especially high mark-up and return for their services. I first dealt with them when Jay received his motorized chair and his hospital bed. Over the course of several years, I regularly received notices from Medicare that they were paying for both pieces of equipment. Then the notices stopped, since both bed and chair had been paid for in full. However, in the case of the medical suppliers, this does not mean that one "owns" these aids but only that they had been paid for. When no longer in use, these must be returned. When the time came to return both, they were immediately reclaimed. Subsequently, I received a surprising notice from Medicare that they had *again* paid the suppliers over sixteen hundred dollars for the chair but had sensibly denied a second payment for the bed. I wrote to Medicare asking why they had paid twice for the chair, but, of course, received no answer. Medicare keeps a low profile by not being able to be contacted at any of its many locations, nor does it ever answer mail.

My memories of annoyance with suppliers ranged over a few other incidents. On reviewing bills for "supplies," I noticed that I was being charged $18.37 for a quart of normal salt solution, which I could have made on my back burner for under ten cents. I didn't contest this because "the suppliers" seem to be a large, more or less interconnected group networked all over the country and I was loathe to tangle with them. The following month, however, the price of the same quart of normal salt solution had risen to $27.78. I gathered that there was a great run on salt that month! (The refusal to round out prices to the nearest dollar was, I believe, begun by Medicare in its payment of doctors. The practice caught on because it seemed to indicate just how precise and accurate the cost of medical services were.)

Jay had arrived in Pennsylvania in the last week of September of 1989. In November our New York suppliers sent a bill for the month of October. I called and informed them that we had not used their services in October and that we had already paid the Pennsylvania suppliers for these. Nonetheless, they insisted that I owed the October bill on some obscure contractual grounds. I replied that I knew of no such contract. They then threatened to take the matter to a lawyer should I fail to pay. I invited them to do so since I would not pay a bill for services I had not received. I heard no more from them. I had won that one, but not without expending much time and energy.

Then I recalled my struggle to obtain a nurse who was legally empowered to manage the feeding machine during weekends. Of course, "the suppliers" had one. The cost, paid directly to them, was a hundred dollars a day. By accident I discovered that the person was paid but sixty dollars a day! But more than that, I discovered that the forty-dollar-a-day fee to the suppliers for getting her the job never came to an end. The nurse owed them forty dollars a day for every day worked, even if the job lasted a year! Quite unlike employment agencies, which have a limit on the fee they can charge an employee for securing the person a job, "the suppliers" obviously had no such limit. The twenty-five-cent phone call to me seems to have brought "the suppliers" a handsome return.

Now that Jay again needed a fancy bed, I thought it would be wise to just buy one. These cost anywhere from three thousand dollars a month rental for the pressure-*removing* beds to the thirteen hundred and fifty dollars we spent in Pennsylvania for the pressure-*relieving* bed (an air mattress with an air pump attached). In the fifteen months Jay had been in Pennsylvania, I had already spent some twenty thousand dollars on such beds and it seemed time to bring this perpetual drain on our savings to an end. Once and for all I would finish off the savings and have the use of the bed as long as he lived.

Now this is not the kind of expense one *plans* to incur. Not realizing what I was getting into, I had gotten involved in supplying these beds for Jay and indeed, they had been of great help in beating back the bedsores. But once "in" there seems to be little way "out." However, despite many calls across the country in search of a price quote on the complete cost of the bed, I never did receive an answer. The promises to return my calls with an answer never materialized. From "the supplier's" point of view it was better that I pay for the bed five times over than that I pay for it once. The only article I have ever seen on the matter of "the suppliers" was a recent one on the flip side of this coin. It recounted evidence that doctors were being paid off to order wheelchairs and motorized lift-chairs for the spritely elderly who were too busy playing golf to sit! So much of the cost of profit-taking here was charged directly to Medicare. There were times when I speculated on just how long it would take the suppliers to deplete Medicare funds entirely.

Considering the difficulties I have had in caring for Jay, it is no wonder that a rising chorus of voices is demanding aid for families faced with long-term care. When Medicare was conceived, the need for such care was minimal and manageable. Patients simply died and this was a factor in shaping the legislation. But every advance in medicine brought the further need for financial help with delayed-dying, which was coming into clearer focus. Middle-class America is taking the brunt of this medical bill.

Needless to say, financial stress produces another psychological mountain to climb. Gradually the wish grows that the patient would die—without pain and fear to be sure—but that he or she would put an end both to his or her empty "life" and to the worries and constrictions suffered by the caregivers. The wish that someone would die is sometimes couched in the euphemistic form of "He has suffered enough," in order to evade a direct confrontation with one of our most insistent prohibitions. Even the variation of this wish into "We have *both* suffered enough" fails to put the taboo to rest. Neither form of the wish succeeds in obscuring the fact that we wish someone dead to relieve our burdens. The climb becomes still more rocky and the footing more treacherous when one appeals to the fact that there is nothing left for the victim to enjoy and no "quality" to the living. Should I, or even can I, have such wishes for someone else with hope of personal psychological immunity?

The taboo against this sentiment is so strong that I realized I had accepted every technological option in sight to prolong life, even the life of the semi-comatose Jay. The realization that he was using resources all of which might best be put to better advantage for others who had some hope of returning to "life," had no impact on me. I consoled myself that my thoughts about Jay's death were only "wishes."

Then one day our daughter, whose continuous love and admiration for her father never wavered, called to suggest that I try to obtain a court order for removal of the feeding tube. She insisted that she *knew* her father wouldn't want to live under these conditions and that we were *forcing* him to do so. Her message was brief, to the point, and powerful. I agreed with her. We were indeed forestalling the natural inclination of his body to die. But since Jay could not communicate, how could we know what, if anything, he may be wishing? How could we make such a decision with assurance?

Our daughter's message, conveyed with such emotional force, made me wonder whether I should have refused the feeding tube in the first place. Would I have refused it had I known then what I now know? But as I thought about it I realized that I could not have refused the feeding tube, since I would never have shouldered the burden of knowing that I had thereby effectively condemned Jay to death, particularly since, at that time, his flickering mind gave some evidence of a vigorous battle to live.

My thoughts ranged over Jay lying there in bed. I knew he could never recover from the extreme brain damage that repeated clot bombardment of his brain had caused. I knew he could never speak again and that I would never again hear his beautifully soft baritone voice with its precise diction. (The tapes of some of his lectures, which a student had given me and which I had counted on to provide a lasting memory didn't catch any of this either.) And I knew that Jay would never emerge from his constricted position. I knew that, in that position, he could never again sit up either in bed or in a "gerichair" and that he was beyond a wheelchair as a conveyance. If he were ever to feel sunshine again, it could only be from inside a room hospitable enough to provide it, and his did not. I knew that he would never again feel a summer breeze or smell the rich aroma of the Vermont forest that he loved so much. Empathy and pity flowed over my consciousness. And it met head-on with resentment at his fate, at my own anguish, and at the enormous expense that this endless and unrelenting illness had occasioned. The opposing feelings could make no peace with each other and so they alternated in dizzying sequences. To be "of one mind" is a fine energizer; to be "of two minds" incapacitates. Yet this frame of mind accurately reflected Jay's situation of not being alive and yet not being dead. I was both a wife and widow at the same time, with all the cares and worries of both estates, with each role fighting the other.

DECISION MAKING AND THE "RIGHT TO DIE"

All caregivers face decision making with an array of options open for the care of their charges. It is my guess that those who nurse stroke victims not only face a greater frequency of decision making but also make many especially momentous and troublesome ones. The reason is simply that, of all those with debilitating diseases, stroke victims have a greater chance for both temporary as well as long-term remission and are sometimes able to be almost totally and permanently repaired. Speech that is slurred or not understandable can be brought back to near normal with the proper therapy; legs that refuse to walk can relearn how to do so. Stroke holds out the possibility of reprieve from incapacity and therefore there are many procedures and techniques available to bring about this result. Beyond rehabilitative measures, the brain itself tends to battle through to regain control of the body even without the aid of technical intervention and remediation. Therefore, the matter of choosing and deciding on a course of action is of utmost importance to the stroke caregiver.

There are problems with decision making of any kind. The process of weighing options and arriving at a satisfactory solution is beset by pitfalls. First, it is most unlikely that we will face a choice between a clear-cut good and an obvious evil. Were this the case, choosing would be easy. What makes choosing a problem is that there is something of both flavors—some good consequences and some unsatisfactory ones—in any choice. The problem then becomes that of determining just what satisfactory and unsatisfactory results each alternative provides. We then come to the toughest part: needing to assign relative weights or levels of importance to each of the consequences. We are then in a position to make a tentative estimate regarding which alternative has the edge for a particular patient's special needs, hopes, and revulsions. The whole process of evaluating which alternative to take (if any) is subject to omission, and error.

It ought to be obvious that for all of these reasons caregivers should not be urged by impatient medical personnel to make crucial decisions on the spot. Time should be given to consult with others and to think about the consequences of both assent as well as denial. In addition, decisions of any magnitude should not fall solely on a lone spouse, already traumatized by a combination of fear, grief, and uncertainty. Such decisions should benefit from the advice and counsel of a group of persons consisting of those closest to the victim; perhaps a close friend or two, a knowledgeable nurse, and a doctor to answer questions. With this procedure any choice could be thrashed out so some consensus can emerge, thus sparing a spouse from sole responsibility.

Needless to say, if a patient can effectively be brought into any decision-making process, the caregiver can have some idea regarding what the loved one would and would not accept. Unfortunately, when this isn't possible, the caregiver either has to go-it-alone or ask for time to evaluate the situation.

Decisions regarding speech therapy, reading therapy, physical therapy, and occupational therapy very much require the cooperation and eagerness of the patient. If he or she cannot communicate inclinations, caregivers have to be constantly alert to nonverbal reactions and modify their decisions accordingly.

Decisions regarding home care versus nursing home care require a more elaborate and self-searching evaluation, which has to include a frank willingness to undertake home care. Other considerations are, of course, the patient's inclination, temperament, and expectations as well as his or her physical and mental condition. It must also include an estimate of the physical properties of the house with respect to accommodating the patient, and certainly a realistic estimate of the family's financial ability to pay for either option. Medicare does not pay for home care, except for very occasional visits by a nurse and for needed devices, such as hospital beds or lift-chairs. Nor does it pay for drugs (prescription or nonprescription) or sickroom needs.

The last year has seen cutbacks in almost every service that Medicare had at one time covered, whether in whole or in part. Cutbacks during the next few years are now predicted to increase both the number of items no longer covered and the extent of reimbursement for medical costs. Only those on Medicaid can dismiss costs from their decisions since their penalty has already been exacted by having to relinquish just about everything they have ever owned to gain entrance into the program.

Life-or-death decisions are quite another matter. Such decisions typically involve employment of technologically advanced machinery and uncommonly expensive techniques and medications, such as some types of radical cardiac resuscitation to artificially shock a stopped heart into further action, the use of an oxygen tent to carry the pneumonia victim through, the use of a feeding tube to supply nutrition, and even the intensive use of antibiotics to combat life-threatening infection. Each may be considered by some caregivers and patients to be efforts at interfering with the threat of death.

There is overwhelming justification for making every effort to save life. Yet the condition of the patient may modify that conviction. There may be times when it might well be more humane to withhold such aids in favor of permitting the suffering loved one to die a peaceful and painless death by means of sedation and pain-killers. There are those who, because of illness or accident, are doomed to be forever deprived of a life that might be called "human." The person who is comatose, the victim of heart disease for whom surgery or transplant would guarantee only a brief reprieve, the Alzheimer's victims whose loss of brain function is so severe as to render them incapable of self-preservation and who are potentially dangerous to themselves, these are all candidates for removal of life-support. These kinds of personal disasters cause us to wonder whether the victim ought not be permitted to die. Might not the rush to technology be an arrogant attempt to preserve life when nature has said no? In hopeless cases is the mission of mercy the one that says no or yes to death?

Situations of this sort pose an excrutiating dilemma for any caregiver. It is just such situations which force us to confront the questions of whether prolonging life by means of technology is not sometimes a cruelty both to the victim and to the family.

One way to lighten the burden of life-or-death decisions and dilemmas would be the development of hospices for just such victims who can no longer be cared for at home, and who don't belong in hospitals or in expensive nursing homes. We have just such accommodations for those who suffer with incurable and often painful types of cancer, and those condemned to an AIDS (Acquired Immune Deficiency Syndrome) death who are finding hospices slowly responding to their needs. Should we not have hospices for those who have no hope of recovery and who medical technology condemns to a meaningless and elongated nonliving?

Another avenue for relieving the cutting edge of life-or-death decisions would be extensive use of the recently developed "right to die" option. There was a day in the almost recent past when few, if any, life-or-death decisions were made. Disease came and had its unimpeded way while caregivers relied almost exclusively on prayer. Doctors did what they could with a very limited medical arsonal. I can even remember when scarlet fever and pneumonia were dreaded diseases; when polio swept through the land, killing and maiming children and adults; and when those with arterial-coronary diseases drew an automatic death sentence. It has only been in the second half of this century, with its tremendous advances in medical research, technology, instrumentation, and methods, that the doors for medical decision making opened wide.

With these advances came increased control over disease and an expanded ability to keep the processes of life going. And of course, with them, came the soaring cost of medical care. Along with the new, intricate, and expensive machines came new and more expensive medical testing. Doctors could no longer be expected to make "house calls," because they needed a full supply of these machines and tests at their disposal. They began to forget their diagnostic skills, which many of us can remember, and to rely more and more on tests both to confirm their judgment and to put it in more exact mathematical terms. Doctors' offices, hospitals, and nursing homes became increasingly expensive to equip. But once outfitted, they were put to full use. It wasn't very long before the cost of medical care outstripped the ability of the average family to pay. The cost was then shifted to Medicare and to private insurances programs, which, in turn, began to feel the "medflation." And this was not merely because doctors wanted more money, but because they had to have all of this new paraphernalia lest they be outclassed and behind the times. Whether the suppliers of such equipment are of the same mind and character as "the suppliers" I encountered is an open question. But the complaint that doctors use this expensive equipment too frequently and often unnecessarily is probably well taken. If the cost of medical care has "skyrocketed," the engine of that rocket is the advance of medical technology.

"Right to die" options emerged from the recognition that the dying patient no longer has need for elaborate technology, which had served its role by having effectively diagnosed the patient as dying. "Right to die" documents are but a way of getting out from under the heavy use of technology and asking instead for peace, quiet, and a fair dose of tender loving care. It has been only in the last ten years or so that the rights of a person to reject available medical options came into prominence. Did patients really want to maintain a limited existence attached to a feeding tube or a respirator? Were patients and their families willing to accept a horribly crippled condition or one in which the mind had already expired? Were we willing to let our loved ones lead empty and servile lives, completely dependent on the care of others? Do we want to live a humiliating and degrading existence?

As the chorus of nos swelled, the demand for a legal right-to-die document increased. Should'nt everyone have some say regarding the kind and quality of life he or she would accept? Whose life was it, anyway? All over the country grassroots groups began asking for and even demanding such rights. A legal instrument was sought to replace the time-honored personal option of rational suicide, which, of course, assumes a competent victim.

While the growing acceptance of a legal "right to die" or "Living Will" option does not seem to impinge directly on what I like to call the "fateful decisions," which many caregivers are called upon to make, it surely does so indirectly. Both decisions presuppose an implicit right to refuse treatment. The social acceptance of the right to determine how one should die loosens up and possibly may even free the right to refuse other kinds of treatment.

However, the two types of "refusal" options have some very crucial differences. The Living Will is made in advance of crisis and is activated by each individual who chooses to have such a document drawn up. Furthermore, it involves no risk since it becomes effective when death is already an imminent certainty. In contrast, "fateful decision" options are made by the caregiver, not the victim, and are typically made on very little notice. Beyond this, they involve a life-or-death gamble. One possible result of such a decision is that the patient might die, thus making the decision maker the responsible party to the disaster.

My first fateful decision for Jay occurred when I was invited to sign a "do not resuscitate" order, which I unhesitatingly signed. Lacking a Living Will for Jay and knowing only that he deeply feared death, I had to take cues from his own body's responses. My reasoning was that many of Jay's most valued abilities had been damaged beyond repair. In addition, he now had life-threatening pneumonia. If, in addition to all of this, his heart would also stop of its own accord, it seemed to me that he was expressing his visceral response to these compound physical afflictions.

My second fateful decision occurred when I was confronted with three options regarding Jay's inability to swallow properly during the several bouts of pneumonia. Option one was to do nothing: death by pneumonia would be inevitable. The second option was to sustain Jay by means of intravenous hydration, thus guaranteeing him a long, drawn-out death by starvation. Only the third choice, the implantation of a feeding tube, seemed humane. I selected the least offensive option as against the yet worse. And I agonized that I might have selected a treatment Jay may not have wanted had he had some input.

Again, I based my judgment on evidences from his body. I gave assent to the feeding tube because his ability to utilize food was still active. What had failed was Jay's mechanical ability to deliver food safely to his stomach because his swallowing was impaired by paralysis. Once the need to swallow was bypassed, his body was able to utilize food and therefore it was still willing to accept the option of life.

However, these two decisions did differ in one very important respect. The do-not-resuscitate choice was made with more or less adequate knowledge of the likely consequences, while the feeding tube option was accepted with a profound ignorance of the many important consequences it harbored. I did not know that feeding machines were difficult to keep in good working order, that tending them was a twenty-four-hour-a-day job, or that the efficient care of Jay's bedsores would be compromised by his attachment to the machine. I surely didn't know that New York State law forbade hiring anyone other than a Licensed Practical Nurse or a Registered Nurse for management of a feeding machine. I also did not know the difficulty in obtaining a qualified nurse for home duty or that the cost of such a service was prohibitive.

There were two important gaps in my information with respect to the three options given to me regarding the feeding tube. Only subsequently did I ask myself whether the doctor was giving me a *genuine* choice. Was the option of rejecting the feeding tube and relying solely on intravenous hydration but a temporary accommodation offered by a sympathetic doctor in order to give me more time to become accustomed to the idea of enteral feeding? Could or would the hospital administration veto any choice I might make that would allow Jay to starve to death while under its care? Of course, I could have taken him home and selected either option. Or could I? Assuming I could have discharged Jay, what were the odds that an interested onlooker (and there were many) would be incited to bring legal action against me for lack of appropriate care?

A patient's right to refuse treatment, let alone a caregiver's, is an intensely troublesome ethical/legal issue that has been at the center of much controversy, and which, to date, has not been resolved. Such decisions seem to rest either on private religious commitment or on personal inclination. As a result, principles for directing our actions are extremely difficult for a diverse society to agree upon.

The second gap in my information was ignorance of the fact that once the decision was made to implant a feeding tube, nothing short of a court order could reverse it. I am puzzled when these two examples of fateful decisions are juxtaposed. Despite the difficulties in achieving broad social approval with respect to such courses of action, the do-not-resuscitate decision seems to have gained it, with the help of well-defined rights, while the equally momentous feeding-tube decision has had no such legal basis. Legal attention and protection of both parties concerned seems to have been given to the do-not-resuscitate choice but not to the feeding-tube choice, even though both of these involve a refusal to accept treatment. Shouldn't the latter choice be afforded the same protection for both patient and spouse that the former rightfully offers?

If this decision dilemma were not muddled enough, I had yet to confront still another, which our daughter posed. Why was I so willing to sign an order not to resuscitate yet I was unwilling to take action to have the feeding tube removed? Both choices were refusals of treatment and both involved opting for Jay's death. On what grounds, therefore, could I support one and reject the other?

My only answer to this puzzle was the fact that science and religion, for so long historical enemies, have now joined forces in agreeing on the importance of human life. Science is convinced that human life is important enough to warrant ceaseless efforts to medically understand it and hence to be able to preserve, protect, and sustain it. Religion is likewise convinced that human life has incalculable worth. But while science proudly brought the weaponry to fight against its loss, religion brings the unshakable conviction that "Only God can giveth and only God can taketh away." Together, they have posed an insuperable dilemma for caregivers. Such debates should make it obvious that a Living Will is a much-needed instrument for relieving the caregiver of impossible decisions.

The Living Will of today is the first step in firming up our right over our own bodies and our own fate. In the bargain, it takes some of the burden of blind decision making off the shoulders, head, and heart of the caregivers. It has been accepted as a legal instrument by most, but by no means all states. Since matters of life and death are so deeply entangled with diverse religious beliefs, it is difficult to get unanimity on the matter.

However, lack of universal support is not the main problem with Living Wills. While they have done much good, they fail, I think, in what they perceive the decision to be. Living Wills simply list equipment and procedures the employment of which their makers can veto. Of course, one might have a special antipathy to a respirator or a feeding machine owing to some previous event or experience. Distaste of this kind needs to be recognized and respected. Apart from this consideration, I don't believe that the "right to die" documents ask the right questions. It seems to me that the heart of the matter lies in just what capacities are so central to a person's life that he or she would not want to live without them. What abilities are so enjoyed (be it physical mobility, communication, use of hands, reading and writing etc.) that the person would feel his or her quality of life severely compromised by their absence? In short, what does the person most value in living? Given this information, a rough estimate can be made of just what illnesses, actions, and procedures could most seriously challenge the person's sense of the worth.

There is yet another flaw in the way Living Wills are drawn up. No medical device or procedure can be evaluated apart from a total picture of both an individual's healthy life and the extent of any present disabilities. A feeding tube cannot be evaluated in isolation from the total physical picture. For example, it is one thing not to want a feeding tube if other physical ailments involve spending the rest of one's life in bed, looking at the ceiling. It is another thing if, in spite of the tube, one is able to return to some share of those activities identified as central to personal fulfillment.

Individuals attach different values to various activities and capacities irrespective of the machines being used to keep them alive. Such value questions should be answered in Living Wills. It might be useful for those who contemplate such a will to write a few sentences on what they most enjoy and why. Possibly they could draw up a table of their value choices, rank-ordering them from least to most valuable. Obviously, answers to such questions will resist becoming part of a computer database. They need to be personally expressed by future patients, whose proxies will rely on these insights when called upon to make difficult medical decisions on behalf of the patient.

There is one final issue regarding the impending death of a patient who is still conscious and aware. One of my friends lay dying with cancer of the spine that had migrated throughout her body. She said, "I am glad that you came today since I don't think I will be conscious tomorrow. Up to this point I have been able to be interested in the world and to relate to my friends. I have been able to be a person. But now the pain has become so great that I can no longer be human. I have asked them to anesthetize me so that I can peacefully die."

The message left a scarring imprint. It reminded me of a movie I saw long ago about an island population in the path of an oncoming hydrogen bomb. The government mercifully supplied its population with suicide pills to be used at each person's discretion if and when it was felt to be necessary. That move transformed the ultimate decision, and the means to carry it out, into a personal choice. Perhaps we should allow some type of solution like this for those who would request it, just in case they are yet able to use it if they wish.

The great triumph of both stories is that human beings were able to determine for themselves when and under what conditions their lives would end. The Living Will is a start—perhaps a first chapter.

Jay, who has been on the front lines of this battle for so long, had never provided me with any guidelines for the type of decisions I have had to make on his behalf. And he now resides in Pennsylvania, a state whose way of understanding the worth of life is closer to the religious vision than to the scientific one. He and his life have therefore not reached their last chapter. He remains inert, semi-comatose, chained to a machine, bound to a body no longer able to sustain its own life and imprisoned in a mind now in semi-darkness, no longer able to comprehend its plight.

On the other hand, God didn't do it. I, the caregiver, did it. For love of him, I had committed a dying man to a feeding tube. I had condemned a beautiful, talented human being to a nonhuman, vegetative existence for the indefinite future!

Afterword

It was late: ten minutes after midnight on the day when spring of 1991 was to arrive. The phone rang. The soft voice of Jay's Pennsylvania doctor said, "The professor died about twenty-five minutes ago."

I sat motionless, silently asking Jay: How did it feel? Did it hurt? Were you frightened? Did you encounter the dark tunnel with the bright light at the end, as reported by those who have been said to have returned after a few moments of being "dead"? Or, as the ancient Greeks believed, have you already embarked on the boat that sailed down the river Lethe, the river of forgetfulness?

Our daughter recently had an unusual and internationally flavored wedding-by-candlelight. The program stated that the music for the couple's processional, the recessional, and all of the organ pieces throughout the ceremony were a tribute to her father's love of Baroque classical music.

At the end of the ceremony, an American Indian statement of the meaning of marriage was read:

"Now there are two of you but neither of you shall be cold
because you will keep one another warm.
"Now there are two of you but neither of you shall be lonely
because you will keep one another company.
"Now there are two of you and there is but one life between
you. . . ."

That was *indeed* what I had lost—the "one life" between us! But, as if in compensation, I had also richly shared the lengthy dying that ended that life.

DATE DUE

MAR 27 2002			
MAR 2 6 2002			
GAYLORD			PRINTED IN U.S.A.